Sobriety

The Ultimate Guide to Successful Recovery

(How to Get Sober From Home Without Leaving Your Family)

Cecile Rankin

Published By **Oliver Leish**

Cecile Rankin

All Rights Reserved

Sobriety: The Ultimate Guide to Successful Recovery (How to Get Sober From Home Without Leaving Your Family)

ISBN 978-1-7388267-1-1

No part of this guidebook shall be reproduced in any form without permission in writing from the publisher except in the case of brief quotations embodied in critical articles or reviews.

Legal & Disclaimer

The information contained in this ebook is not designed to replace or take the place of any form of medicine or professional medical advice. The information in this ebook has been provided for educational & entertainment purposes only.

The information contained in this book has been compiled from sources deemed reliable, and it is accurate to the best of the Author's knowledge; however, the Author cannot guarantee its accuracy and validity and cannot be held liable for any errors or omissions. Changes are periodically made to this book. You must consult your doctor or get professional medical advice before using any of the suggested remedies, techniques, or information in this book.

Upon using the information contained in this book, you agree to hold harmless the Author from and against any damages, costs, and expenses, including any legal fees potentially resulting from the application of any of the information provided by this guide. This disclaimer applies to any damages or injury caused by the use and application, whether directly or indirectly, of any advice or information presented, whether for breach of contract, tort, negligence, personal injury, criminal intent, or under any other cause of action.

You agree to accept all risks of using the information presented inside this book. You need to consult a professional medical practitioner in order to ensure you are both able and healthy enough to participate in this program.

Table Of Contents

Chapter 1: Alcohol In Our Culture 1

Chapter 2: Understanding Your Habits And Needs 20

Chapter 3: First Steps To Freedom 48

Chapter 4: The Approach 73

Chapter 5: Psychological Focus 108

Chapter 6: Social Focus 122

Chapter 7: Getting Sober 154

Chapter 8: Bottle Divers 177

Chapter 1: Alcohol In Our Culture

"First you take a drink, then the drink takes a drink, then the drink takes you."
– F. Scott Fitzgerald

Alcohol has long been regarded as a candy remedy within the direction of human facts. The fermented beverage originated from fruit, greens, and even honey in the Neolithic era, evolving into what we now recognise as vodka, whiskey, brandy, vermouth, cognac, beer, and greater. Chemically known as "ethyl" alcohol or ethanol, it's been organized and ate up thru humans for at least 7,000 years of human history. From the southeast of Asia to ancient Egypt, alcohol predates maximum of recorded history, with China considered to be its area of beginning. The Babylonians worshiped a wine goddess in 2,seven-hundred B.C., on the identical time as the Greeks kept away from alcohol consumption of their earliest literature. The reality stays that alcohol has been a part of popular way of life all at some point of the globe considering the truth that time immemorial.

Indigenous peoples of the Americas developed grain-based alcohol inside the form of "chicha," a beverage organized from fermented corn, grapes, and apples. Alcohol served as a medicinal additive in the 1600s and, within the 18th century, it changed into termed "spirits" in acknowledgment of its alchemic houses.

The mid 18th century witnessed a reform inside the consumption of alcohol. What turned into as quickly as used as an additive to remedy changed into now desired as an after-hours beverage whilst the British Parliament recommended using grain to offer distilled spirits. This brought about a skyrocketing call for for gin, with its intake peaking at 18 million gallons. Great Britain became a country that recommended eating.

In the early 19th century, alcohol modified into in the end recognized as an lousy drink, and the eating of it had to be discouraged. Hence, the emergence of the Temperance Movement. Later on, this movement superior into zero tolerance closer to alcohol, which end up heartily rejected in America. It wasn't until 1920 that the united states took felony motion to restrict the change of alcohol on an worldwide scale, but even that had little impact. The ban—known as Prohibition—didn't save you people from making, shopping for, promoting, or consuming alcohol and gave upward push to the illegal alcohol exchange within the Nineteen Thirties. Prohibition in America ended in 1933.

Today, about 15 million Americans are appeared as alcoholics.

Reflection, Imitation, Social Experiences
In a society that facilitates alcohol use, social effect is wherein all of it begins offevolved. Studies screen the correlation amongst alcoholism and its "partners in crime," i.E., the social conditions that inspire eating. Having a drink with pals plays a huge function inside the unfold of alcoholism. The have an effect on of human beings over their friends suggests that

the selection to be socially common can bring about alcoholism (Dallas et al., 2014; Larsen, Engels, Granic, & Overbeek, 2009; Larsen, Engels, Souren, Granic, & Overbeek, 2010). In addition, those studies discovered that the type of beverages in step with man or woman will boom because the type of humans in a hard and rapid of pals will boom. However, a predisposition to alcoholism is the primary wrongdoer. Recent findings advocate an character's opportunity of indulgence is more large once they've already tailored to social situations that include liberal consuming of alcohol. In much less complicated terms, human beings are much more likely to enjoy social bonding via consuming with others in the event that they've been delivered to this concept growing up. (Creswell et al., 2012).

Imitating others thru consuming alcohol is an try to sell bonding amongst people at social sports that have ingesting as a ordinary workout. Looking at this each different manner, it's in particular awkward now not to eat on the equal time as all people spherical you is ingesting, and it's the identical with eating alcohol. From a systematic factor of view, consuming may be a form of imitation, but eating is associated more with people on the lookout for validation among their friends. Social recognition is what the "human beings pleaser" seeks, and eating makes this appear greater to be had.

Alcohol Use Around Us
From an accompaniment to Mediterranean cuisine to "happy hour," alcohol has end up a staple in just about every way of existence. Its use is turning into greater great, driven by way of using misconceptions that thrive in our collective societies. As we've visible, alcohol modified into as quick as extensively considered as some thing wholesome. "A glass of wine an afternoon maintains the scientific health practitioner away" modified into the excuse that indulgers may use because there's evidence that positive kinds of alcohol (crimson wine, in maximum times) assist save you coronary coronary heart disease. However, this claim emerge as rejected with the aid of a

worldwide observe posted in The Lancet that analyzed the outcomes of alcohol on purchasers in 195 nations over 16 years. The effects concluded that the effects of alcohol intake greatly outweigh the benefits. So-known as "moderate consuming" has many negative repercussions, with an improved danger of most cancers being among them.

"The maximum regular quantity of alcohol is none," changed into the choice of this studies. The have a take a look at analyzed a huge shape of damaging consequences associated right now to alcohol intake, from drunken the use of incidents to self-harm and greater. What was critically demanding turned into the huge screen that almost 10% of early deaths in humans inside the 15-to-40 nine age institution had been because of alcohol consumption.

The Alcohol Illusion

Let's admit it. Alcohol doesn't flavor top notch, it doesn't benefit you in any manner, and it fees lots too. So why is it that we nonetheless have a tendency to accomplice alcohol with "right instances?" The inclination inside the path of indulgence begins offevolved pretty early, and at the same time as surely absolutely everyone shun the concept of early ingesting, it's encouraged at the equal time as we emerge as adults. The damage it creates is the same, whether or now not the drinker is a teen or an person, so the double preferred isn't handiest ironic but illogical.

The belief that alcohol enhances the pride of other sports isn't always something more than an phantasm. The concept that ingesting alcohol makes you appear more brand new and lets in you to loosen up extra is a myth. A drink of heterosexual alcohol is some thing but a laugh, and combining the venom with sweeter nectars best mask the awfulness. If you're ingesting greater than instances every week, you're already at the dependancy spectrum.

If you attempt and reduce your intake, you'll experience the withdrawal outcomes—which often leads you to have genuinely "one more drink," which in brief relieves your distress. You inform yourself that end up the "last," however that is in which the in no way-finishing circle of defeat starts. Just a glass will now not satisfy you. Before you are aware about it, you've been sucked deep into the vicious cycle of alcoholism, illness, broken relationships, career loss, and a awful recognition.

When you understand you want extra alcohol than you used to, you have got got have been given a problem. This is the primary and maximum critical step. Admitting there's a hassle is the hardest factor for maximum alcoholics, but once you acquire that milestone, you're already on the direction to restoration.

Everyone You Know Drinks Alcohol, So How Come it's Just You Who Has a Problem?
Putting your self under the microscope and doing "evaluation to paralysis" is reachable for those in denial. You try and determine out why every body else doesn't appear to have a hassle with consuming, and also you do, however you need to apprehend that "everybody else" isn't

your hassle. You're liable for your body and your fitness, no longer theirs. In precise words, you want to "thoughts your very own industrial business corporation." Comparing our terrible conduct to the ones of others is a incorrect method first of all. There's no competition proper here, so why do you want to assess your studies with those of others?

Different our our our bodies have extraordinary metabolism charges, so the results of alcohol range from man or woman to man or woman. However, it's an addictive substance regardless of who the person is. Statistics display the repercussions of alcohol abuse don't discriminate in opposition to age, race, or gender. Denial isn't the way to transport.

Notice when you have any of those symptoms and signs and signs of alcohol dependancy:

-   You're dropping bear in mind of the type of images you're gulping down.
-   You feel ill greater regularly after eating.

- You're no longer as touchy to the outcomes of alcohol, and it fails to offer you a buzz.
- The yearning is getting out of hand.
- Life is an awful lot a lot much less a laugh.
- You're turning into greater aggressive.
- You want to drink to get thru the day.
- You're becoming reckless.
- You keep getting sick.
- Other regions of your existence are beginning to undergo.

From a systematic factor of view, research has confirmed that the body's metabolism determines the outcomes of alcohol. The metabolism of alcohol, in flip, is significantly precipitated with the aid of the usage of genetic elements, environmental factors, and the quantity of alcohol ate up. In a nutshell, alcoholism is advocated through the elements mentioned in advance in the economic ruin— the predisposition to drinking alcohol, social imitation, and lifestyles research.

What Is Alcoholism?

The biochemistry of ethyl alcohol inside the body is a complicated era. Alcohol become the 7th predominant purpose of loss of lifestyles globally in 2016, which brought about an updated evaluation of its molecular biology thru the use of The Lancet (1873a). Metabolized predominantly through using the liver, the effects of alcohol first of all take place in the huge annoying device—therefore its impact on social conduct. However, its no longer on time consequences are even more excessive.

Alcohol is metabolized via the use of numerous pathways. The maximum extensive techniques include enzymes—dehydrogenase (ADH) and aldehyde dehydrogenase (ALDH)—which resource in breaking down ethanol. ADH converts alcohol to acetaldehyde, a pretty toxic substance that's been diagnosed as a carcinogen. Later inside the approach, acetaldehyde is metabolized into acetate, which, in turn, is broken down into water and carbon dioxide. You may additionally additionally take delivery of as real with that due to the fact the save you merchandise of alcohol metabolism are surely water and carbon dioxide, it would be harmless, but there's lots extra to it than that. The toxicity involved within the approach takes a toll at the liver. Not simply that, alcohol additionally damages the pancreas, the mind, the heart, and the essential disturbing tool. As cited formerly, alcohol is implicated in liver most cancers.

What Does It Mean to Get Drunk? What Does It Mean to Have a Hangover?

It takes the liver from one to 2 hours to metabolize alcohol into its constituent compounds. When the range of beverages exceeds the liver's overall performance, we witness the "drunken" united states taking impact. A hangover, which typically happens after a night time time time of excessive alcohol consumption, is regularly due to dehydration and electrolyte imbalances that purpose headache, nausea, stomach cramps, moderate sensitivity, dizziness, horrible sleep, inflammation, and vomiting.

Legally, being "drunk" takes area even as the blood-alcohol content material (BOC) is 0.08 or better, with something near 0.40 typically being deadly. The drunken country may be seen in an individual's coordination, stability, speech, and reflexes. An excessively excessive blood-alcohol degree will restrict an person's functionality to look, stay wide awake, and focus while wanted. Drinking large quantities of alcohol in a quick time period will get worse the outcomes and can reason alcohol poisoning, coma, or maybe loss of lifestyles.

What Is an Alcoholic?
The phrase "alcoholic" can also bring to thoughts the image of a sad, barely overweight, blue-collar male with a bottle of beer who's going thru a mid-life catastrophe. However, it isn't continuously easy to become privy to an alcoholic. Alcoholism could have an impact on human beings from all walks of life—from teens to the aged, rich or bad. Celebrities with notable seems and wealthy careers like Anna Nicole Smith and John Barrymore misplaced

their lives to alcoholism, so appearances can in reality be deceiving.

The very first tell-tale symptoms of an alcoholic encompass the subsequent crimson flags:

- Appearing to be in a kingdom of intoxication most of the time.
- No constraints on eating, be it at work or after hours.
- The urge to drink will increase, and so does the amount or electricity of the liquor.
- A tired appearance and a cranky mind-set.
- Inefficiency.
- A loss of hobby in everyday life.
- Being unhappy and depressed maximum of the time.
- Dishonest and secretive.

An individual displaying some of the ones symptoms and signs may be an alcoholic. Still, given that society has stigmatized the word as a few factor humiliating, we might chorus from terming an individual with a ingesting hassle an alcoholic to spare the sufferer shame or maybe scandal. Because of the massive availability of alcohol at quite an entire lot any social occasion and its attractiveness with the aid of our society, it appears unfair in rate alcoholism on its sufferers.

Some colleges of notion select the "difficult love" approach of shaming the alcoholic if you need to help the person abstain from consuming, however this technique hardly ever works. A guilt-ridden intoxicated man or woman might be to indulge even greater inside the habit, and in excessive cases, they'll even contemplate suicide. The burden of being an "alcoholic" is heavy, and blaming the sufferer isn't useful. A proactive approach is wanted, with counseling being the number one step.

Alcohol Damage
Addiction takes various lengths of time to grow to be installation relying at the man or woman, however what remains everyday is the tolerance to alcohol that builds up, which takes place in anybody who beverages frequently. A specific person can be extra vulnerable to the harmful results of alcohol, while some different

is probably lots less so. Over time, ordinary alcohol intake reasons an imbalance in gamma-aminobutyric acid (GABA), a neurotransmitter liable for controlling impulsivity. Not quality that, alcoholism disrupts the steadiness of glutamate, every other neurotransmitter that's chargeable for sending indicators to specific forms of cells in the body.

Dopamine is likewise a neurotransmitter, and on the equal time as dopamine levels inside the mind increase, we revel in pleasure. Over time, the thoughts will become addicted to the discharge of dopamine, that's one of the roots of addiction. The body calls for an increasing number of dopamine launch to experience the euphoria of delight.

If someone consumes massive portions of alcohol frequently, their tolerance can boom, and the frame calls for additonal alcohol to obtain the desired effect. This will, purpose the development of lifestyles-threatening illnesses like most cancers of the breast, mouth, esophagus, voice field, colon, rectum, and throat. Other conditions may also encompass high blood stress, liver ailment, chronic digestive troubles, and extra.

The Cost of Drinking

The Centers for Disease Control and Prevention (CDC) estimate that alcoholism charges the us monetary tool $249 billion each one year. This breaks proper right down to $28 billion in healthcare prices, $179 billion in loss of workplace productiveness, $25 billion in alcohol-associated crook justice times, and $thirteen billion in injuries and collisions.

On a smaller scale, an man or woman can pay round $10 in step with drink in a bar or ingesting set up order, depending at the emblem of alcohol and the way upscale the venue in which it's being offered. Seldom does an individual at a bar or restaurant prevent at a single drink. According to CDC stats, a male purchaser commonly beverages 4 to fourteen liquids normal with week, and a mean lady will eat four to seven alcoholic beverages consistent with week. The rate of alcoholism doesn't give up there. Broken relationships, DUI tickets, healthcare fees, hobby loss, and out of place possibilities make alcoholism one of the most expensive lousy behavior.

In total, alcohol-associated conditions and infection are anticipated to value NHS England approximately £3.Five billion every year, so it's no longer handiest a extreme problem inside the USA. Alcoholism is a global hassle, and its real-time prices seem in healthcare, own family existence, efficiency at the pastime, and extraordinary components. These can't be successfully measured, so it's not viable to region a greenback quantity on its outcomes in those regions. All the extra annoying is that an alarming percentage of alcohol use infection (AUD) patients sooner or later lodge to drug abuse, making alcohol abuse straight away associated with drug abuse. By digging deeper into all the mishaps and losses associated with capsules, you might be capable of understand to a degree the quantity of harm alcohol reasons, economically and in any other case.

Chapter 2: Understanding Your Habits And Needs

"The preliminary journey in the course of sobriety is a sensitive balance among belief into one's preference for get away and abstinence from one's addiction." — Debra L. Kaplan

The Basics of Habits

Abraham Maslow, an American psychiatrist, described psychotherapy as having the detail of "self" as its cornerstone. With the appearance of the modern-day-day "self-actualization" topic, Millennials and their contrary numbers in Gen Z and Gen X have perverted this precept into an excuse for a night out binge ingesting. This is how alcoholic behavior begin.

Bad conduct originate from four fundamental steps: the cue, the craving, the response, and the reward. With eating, the cue is initiated at the same time as you deliberately have been given right down to drink. With a few aspect as to be had and addictive as alcohol, the sample can set in pretty with out problems, and earlier than you realize it, the craving phase starts offevolved. The response is while you fulfill the ones cravings, and the reward is the sensation of fake contentment you get at the same time as you reach a kingdom of intoxication. A New York Times bestseller, The Atomic Habit, defined life due to the fact the sum of our conduct. If consuming has come to be a dependancy, what does that recommend on your life? Now there's some meals for idea.

Your Most Fundamental Needs

Looking at Maslow"s Hierarchy of Needs, we comprehend that alcohol doesn't in shape into the pyramid everywhere in any respect, so it's not a "want" first of all. The pinnacle of the pyramid is "self-actualization," which inspires innovation, creativity, growth, and abundance—none of which alcohol permits. To advantage the top of the hierarchy, the decrease-down dreams have to be met. Physical goals which includes meals, secure haven, sleep, and clothing are step one, followed via manner of way of the second one tier in the hierarchy, protection desires. Safety goals doesn't truly talk with safety from robbers and losses. They moreover ought to do with emotional balance, properly-being, and economic safety—all subjects that alcohol can rob you of.

The 1/3 tier is the need to be cherished and belong. Family bonds and social sports occupy this slot. Alcohol is the precept wrongdoer in ruining own family bonds and can even carry out aggression in an man or woman. Sharing your eating interest at a bar with a friend may also additionally fulfill the dreams of being loved and belonging for those few moments, however this isn't a wholesome or sustainable manner for getting the ones.

The fourth step in the pyramid is "esteem needs." This refers to an individual's want for self-recognize, acknowledgment, and appreciation for their achievements and existence. Alcohol extensively hinders this element of one's existence. Being an alcoholic robs you of yourself-recognize and, ultimately, your social reputation as properly. It undermines your capability and blocks you from undertaking your goals.

Your Needs as an Alcohol Drinker
Alcoholism is all another time length for alcohol abuse. Once we widely known we're an alcoholic, we're able to get on the direction to healing. This is wherein wonderful modifications begin, however the alcoholic need to first look at their needs as an character with AUD. Those desires ought to revolve spherical abstaining from alcohol.

Let's talk the possible techniques an alcoholic might in all likelihood use to transport into abstinence:

- The DIY technique: Before you inn to rehab, you could constantly start at domestic. Remove all alcohol from your private home. If it's no longer resultseasily in benefit, you're more likely to govern your ingesting conduct.

- Address your demons: There may be underlying problems in your surroundings that motive you into grabbing a drink. Are you in a poisonous courting? Does your process play a function in stressing you out to the point in that you often feel you need a drink? Are you affected by melancholy, trauma, or special intellectual contamination? Compromised highbrow fitness can play a massive position in alcoholism.

- Stay proactive: Keeping numbers of supportive human beings or groups stored in your cellular phone is a vital step. Free data about quitting ingesting is available on the net and in e-books to help you apprehend alcoholism.

- Notice your styles. A pattern refers to a country of thoughts that leads an individual into a selected behavior. Study your styles. If you be aware a pattern, it is going to be much less difficult so you can dispose of what triggers you into grabbing a drink. Moreover, a counselor will let you parent out a plan which will prevent you from falling lower again into an bad sample. In times that require deeper inner art work, cognitive behavioral therapy can assist human beings regain their stability.

- Support: It's usually smart to short your without delay own family about an dependancy hassle. Professional packages can help with restoration with the resource of supplying company treatment, hobby remedy, and further.

Understanding Why You Drink

As said in advance, the common reasons why people drink embody social reputation, speedy escaping strain, improving delight, and, in a few parents, bringing out the daredevil in them. A observe accomplished at PMC Labs decided that the two number one reasons of heavy eating are terrible reinforcement and terrific reinforcement. The former implies that an man or woman beverages as a coping mechanism to keep away from feelings of hopelessness, sadness, and melancholy. The latter has to do with "letting free" and being greater sociable.

Cahalan et al. (1969) described the 2 unique groups of drinkers in greater detail, indicating that social reasons for drinking had been associated more with lighter drinkers on the equal time as abusive consuming had greater to do with individuals searching out to deal with issues. Nonetheless, the findings guide the concept that social consuming can although cause alcoholism.

This look at found elevated indulgence in the horrific-reinforcement company when they have been confronted with situations that exacerbated their stress, on the identical time as the powerful-reinforcement institution drank greater while socializing more. The two corporations have been in addition broken down into gender, ethnicity, and age. The test determined that grownup men were better able to deal with pressure without overdrinking than have been women. Yet, men are much more likely to be alcoholics than women. The take a look at had a few conflicting effects. The final end have grow to be that any person with a longing for alcohol will supply in to the urge now and then, no matter whether or no longer their purpose is pushed thru bad or powerful reinforcement.

Alcohol, in its essence, is a depressant. Clinically defined as a sedative, it numbs the senses and adjustments an individual's emotional responses.

In moderate of Maslow's Hierarchy of Needs, in which does that depart the AUD victim? What are your reasons for ingesting? You may additionally now not have a reason because dependancy has taken away your potential to pick out your conduct.

Do You Have a Problem with Alcohol?

Before we start to dissect the information of alcohol addiction, allow's first address the elephant in the room: Are you a hassle drinker? If so, are you capable of admit this, or are you in denial? Studies reveal that the recognition of being an alcohol abuser aids surprisingly in an character's restoration. However, a few human beings are really clueless about whether or not or not they've evolved an alcohol addiction. The following questions will assist you find out your reputation regarding alcohol use:

- Do you emerge as drinking greater than you recall to?
- Does your conventional quantity of liquids work the manner they used to?
- Would you as a substitute drink than take pride in a favorite interest or interest?
- Have you tried to quit eating and did not achieve this?
- Do you crave alcohol?
- How a amazing deal time do you spend eating?
- Is eating turning into a problem for the people spherical you?
- Have you gotten into any shape of hassle because of ingesting?
- Has ingesting landed you in dangerous conditions like tickets for DUI or fights?
- Do you suffer withdrawal signs and symptoms at the same time as you refrain from consuming?

Answers to the ones questions will assist show your relationship with alcohol, but a deeper approach from a scientific attitude is needed. Blood tests beneficial aid in assessing whether an individual has been ingesting cautiously for a extended duration. Lab paintings can indicate a decrease in purple blood cells, that could be a symptom of extended alcohol abuse. Testing for carbohydrate-negative transferrin (CDT) can monitor if someone has been ingesting immoderate quantities of alcohol every day or has relapsed after now not consuming for some time. Other assessments may be needed to investigate a binge drinker's liver damage and reduced testosterone tiers in guys.

How Much Do You Drink?
The street to alcoholism is a hard one. From pints to goblets, martini glasses to images, knowledge the quantity of alcohol in a selected drink is a technology in its non-public right. On top of this is the task of keeping score of approaches masses you drink, which can be quite the ordeal. How does the layman even understand how a good deal a "unit" of alcohol

is on the manner to track their consumption? A unit is the diploma delivered in the UK in 1987 to help humans music the amount of alcohol they consume. One unit equals 10 ml or 0.34 fl ozof alcohol—the amount the liver metabolizes in about an hour. In a lot much less complex words, a unit of alcohol want to take about one hour to go away the body.

Keeping score of the quantity of alcohol entering your body can help in identifying whether or not or now not you've got were given had been given alcoholism. It might possibly sound a bit contradictory, for the reason that we said in advance that no quantity of alcohol is stable, however maintaining music of consumption is sometimes the most effective manner for an abuser to wean themselves from their addiction. Apart from that, a 0-tolerance attitude in the direction of liquor is an unrealistic concept for max humans. Keeping tabs at the kind of drinks consumed appears extra realistic if the idea of abstinence appears impossible.

It's been advocated that ladies and men refrain from ingesting greater than 14 devices of alcohol in keeping with week. It's loads greater healthy to spread this intake over severa days in consistent with week instead of imbibing the 14 gadgets in a unmarried flow. If a drinker can reduce their intake from liquids an afternoon to at least one, they're nicely on their manner to refraining from consuming the least bit for two or 3 days. This is how the frame is educated into returning to regular and functioning properly without the each day alcohol dose. There can be withdrawal signs and symptoms, however with this step-down ordinary, they received't be as immoderate.

For all and sundry looking to wean off of alcohol absolutely, be conscious that becoming sober is greater difficult than falling into alcoholism. But keep in mind, whilst the going gets difficult, the hard get going. There might be days in which you'll experience sick to the bone, and there will be times at the same time as you could relapse. Know that this is all a part of the gadget. To shop your treasured existence, there's no one of a kind manner however to accept the minor setbacks and preserve going beforehand along with your plan to be smooth and sober.

What Does it Mean to Stop Drinking Alcohol?

This is the essence of the campaign you've all commenced: What does it suggest in case you save you consuming alcohol? Are you thinking about abstaining from genuinely the drink, or is it a entire life-style you're willing to allow flow of to live sober? There's plenty extra than what meets the eye with alcoholism. Just as alcohol influences people in a wonderful manner, the motives why an man or woman desires to forestall alcohol range from individual to person. For some, it might be to regain the wholesome appearance they as soon as had. For others, they want to avoid the sickening hangover. Others may additionally moreover choice to save you eating for religious or spiritual reasons. Individuals can also moreover even attempt sobriety as a diet regime because of the truth alcohol can lead to weight problems.

The motive you want to give up alcohol need to be crystal clean on your mind as it performs a vital characteristic in your power of will. With some thing as addictive and dangerous as alcohol, the selection to stop ought to be first discussed with a fitness professional. In nearly each u . S . A ., there are authorities corporations to useful resource you with free services and counseling all along your adventure. Quitting alcohol "cold turkey" incorporates crucial dangers for alcoholics, so a expert's supervision is needed to assist the individual through the acute withdrawal phase.

Withdrawal symptoms and signs variety from nausea, trembling, dizziness, sleeplessness, cold sweats, or perhaps coronary heart palpitations to convulsions and hallucinations. These signs and symptoms and signs and symptoms and signs and symptoms can be excessive, and being below near statement can be important for some human beings. A expert also can assist relieve the signs and symptoms with remedy, counseling, and intellectual guide. Programs are designed to allocate a team of experts to assist the character thru this method. Signing up with a aid system to your region is significantly advocated to preserve your sobriety.

Recognizing You Have a Problem
Alcohol abuse can cripple your lifestyles in many processes. The listing is an extended one. Alcoholism can be deadly, and health headaches are sometimes irreversible. With all of the proof of the damage that alcohol can reason and the help to be had to address alcohol abuse, it's although an prolonged avenue from illness to restoration, which calls for a few in-depth assessment. Alcoholism is curable, but the loss of life toll doesn't seem to dwindle.

Information on line explores each element of research however overlooks a critical and obvious element: denial of being an alcoholic. Alcoholics are unwilling to confess that alcoholism locations them in danger of an early dying and plays a super role of their diminishing fitness. Denial prevents individuals from searching for help that would reason restoration, reduces their possibilities of survival, prevents them from gaining manage in their lives, and sends them into a downward spiral. Denial is not uncommon in alcohol abusers—especially individuals who perished from the contamination.

Indulgers may additionally moreover play the blame game pretty well, and that, too, is a form of denial as is rationalizing their dating with alcohol. Instead of falling prey to denial, you need to widely recognized the trouble and admit you're abusing alcohol. Being protective about a terrible addiction only delays your healing. Value your lifestyles, and understand you've got were given a hassle. Once you take shipping of your mistakes, you could begin your journey to restoration.

What Are Your Reasons for Considering Quitting Alcohol?

Once you've commonplace which you have a problem, it's time to slender down the alternatives for the manner to deal with it. What are the reasons you need to prevent consuming? It's typically not because of the fact your scientific doctor or your own family informed you to. Why did you start ingesting? What caused you to are in search of secure haven in alcohol? Was it a catastrophic event that led you to begin ingesting? Was it a relationship? Is consuming a way as a manner to method grief and past trauma? Once you apprehend the reasons for why you drink, you can see how alcoholism become in no way the answer and the way it best made your troubles worse.

Understanding what made you switch to alcohol will assist preserve you on your efforts. In the past severa many years, alcohol use among young adults has extended. According to surveys finished at the request of TeensHealth, one of the essential factors that make contributions to underage consuming is peer stress. The faux promise in mainstream media that eating makes an man or woman "sense better" is each different massive reason for the upward push in alcohol use amongst young adults. Another contributor is an unstable domestic lifestyles essential to alcohol use as a coping mechanism. The reasons for alcohol abuse amongst teenagers are very just like those of adults who abuse alcohol.

Once the motive in the returned of alcoholism is recognized, it can be said. After that, the following step is to understand that sobriety has extra to do together with your thoughts-set than your cravings. If you've got a clean attitude on what you want for your existence, you'll achieve success.

Denial
As stated formerly, "denial" is a extraordinary difficulty that sets you decrease lower returned from recovery. You outright deny you have got a hassle with alcohol, and you're not in a role or unwilling to confess your dependency.

The denial factor is the maximum irritating detail for those handling some exclusive's alcohol abuse hassle. It may additionally motive the individual's guide team to emerge as discouraged. It might also even occur that the problem drinker's pals and family begin to deny there's a hassle. When denial is just too overpowering, the best way out is for the alcoholic to in the end admit they've got a hassle in place of blaming their addiction at the people spherical them, their existence scenario, or "destiny." Common excuses of deniers embody, "He/She ruined my life," "He/She dumped me," "I don't have any unique way out but to drink," or "Alcohol is the only way I can numb the ache." These excuses are usually followed with the useful resource of an arrogant mind-set. A hassle drinker will deny their breath smells of alcohol or deliver a inclined excuse for ingesting: "I bought the bottle of wine for visitors coming over," or "I stopped via using at the pub for a assembly." The extra you confront them, the greater shielding they get. At times, it's clearly the "I'll do as I please" refrain and, at brilliant instances, it's the "Just one drink" track-and-dance. Confrontation is the toughest a part of the gadget. An alcoholic isn't always frequently organized to confess they have got a problem on the same time as faced. At times, even the parents and buddies will be lied to and given excuses.

Sometimes, the sufferer will accept as real with you that they want to forestall, however the truth that they have got no intention of doing this. They'll say, "You're right. From nowadays onwards, I'm now not touching a drop." As quick as you're out of sight, they're off attempting to find a drink. Denial can also even include comparing themselves to a person else with factors like, "George has been consuming all his lifestyles, he's older than I am, and he's doing pretty suitable."

Denial has many faces, but the longer abusers downplay their dependancy, the more the threat of ill health or dying.

You Aren't Alone
Instead of beating across the bush and playing along with your existence, it's essential to confront your addiction, notwithstanding the

fact that it can seem excessive to confess you're an alcoholic. The CDC estimates 4.Five% of men and 2.Five% of girls be afflicted by means of alcoholism, so it's in fact now not definitely you who has a hassle—neither is it your fault. One in each three households in the US has a person in their prolonged social circle who suffers from alcohol abuse. The fact that the ailment stays stigmatized has substantially hindered recognition of it on a mass scale.

Drinking a can of beer is considered a harmless social act, but alcoholism consists of a stigma. Individuals with AUD are below strain to preserve their addiction a mystery, which only fuels denial. Secrets break lives. It's sufficient which you be affected by the usage of alcoholism. You don't need to undergo it by myself. Know that there's typically help if best you acquire out. If you've got a judgmental circle of relatives, strive starting as an awful lot as a pal. Contact a expert if pals aren't information—or are alcohol abusers themselves. Don't experience embarrassed to be troubled through a condition that's plagued humanity for loads of years.

On a greater intention be aware, alcoholism hardly ever takes vicinity in just one family member. Drug dependancy and alcoholism are regularly considered "circle of relatives illnesses." This approach addiction may be contagious—much like social ingesting—even though it's now not viral. Put certainly, alcoholism is much more likely if a near family member is an alcoholic. Frequently, family will attempt to intervene to assist an alcoholic family member, however for the motive that sickness is complex, they're frequently not a success. If you're suffering from alcohol abuse, you have got a more hazard of getting someone round you who's walked the same path. Former sufferers can assist an alcoholic higher because of the fact they apprehend what it's like.

Hitting Rock Bottom

Alcohol use illness is a fitness difficulty on a international scale. Whether it's considered as a social evil or only a terrible addiction, the reality stays that the sickness has wreaked havoc on endless lives. Many human beings laid low with AUD fail to cope with the problem successfully. Research has determined out that "hitting rock backside" is a essential thing in motivating an individual to forestall consuming and hold their life. From the indulger's angle, hitting rock bottom is when they eventually renowned they want assist with their AUD.

What constitutes rock bottom is particular for every character. For a few, it is probably the close to-demise revel in of alcohol poisoning. For others, it may be that their companion walked out on them because of their AUD. Hitting rock bottom has been termed the tipping factor that compels humans to are looking for treatment (Cunningham et al., 1994). However, the phenomenon of "rock bottom" has in no manner been described in terms of particular signs and symptoms and signs and symptoms and signs and symptoms, so the definition stays subjective.

As dangerous as hitting rock bottom may additionally sound, it's helped human beings climb lower lower back as plenty as sobriety. The experience has been normally defined because the alcoholic awakening to the conclusion that one more drink or one greater binge may be their ultimate. They also can see their lifestyles flashing in advance than their eyes and understand that it's now or in no manner. It's at this element that they get crucial about sobriety.

Moderation: One Drink at a Time

As cited in advance, alcohol addiction comes with a price. Even while you decide to remove the demon, it maintains to haunt you with a vengeance. Withdrawal symptoms and signs can go away someone debilitated, and going cold turkey makes the signs and signs and symptoms and symptoms even worse. Heart palpitations, sleeplessness, loss of urge for food, cold sweats, a regular u . S . A . Of tension, convulsions, and shivering are some of the signs an alcoholic may also face of their quest for sobriety.

Consuming alcohol locations you prone to coronary heart sickness, numerous sorts of most cancers, cirrhosis, a compromised first-rate of lifestyles, and masses of DUI tickets. On the alternative hand, stopping drinking can set you up for debilitating withdrawal symptoms. So, in which does that leave you? Seeking to grow to be sober might also at instances have you feeling torn between saving your life or giving up on it altogether. Nonetheless, there's a manner out. The sweet spot in the quest for sobriety is known as "moderation."

The moderation approach is the extra realistic manner to acquire sobriety. Just as stopping excessive exceptional medicinal pills all of sudden has its drawbacks, the equal is real of alcohol. Moderation lets in you to frequently wean off alcohol to allow your frame to slowly adjust to what it's come to be relying on.

For an alcoholic, consuming alcohol even occasionally is as an alternative discouraged. However, an occasional drink is every so often essential for the sake of their nicely-being. While the advocated mild alcohol consumption is restrained to two liquids or fewer a day for men and one drink or fewer an afternoon for women, an addict may need extra or much less of the encouraged slight amount depending on their frame and dependancy state of affairs.

Sobriety

Commonly described as turning a long way from alcoholism, "sobriety" is particularly misunderstood. Although the term refers to complete abstinence from alcohol, it has to do with greater than truely alcohol. Sobriety is, in fact, a change of manner of life. The only measures along the direction to sobriety frequently encompass converting your circle of buddies and your regular hangouts. It's an extensive reforming of your lifestyles and calls for popular willpower.

Sobriety is regularly regarded as freedom from drug abuse, alcohol, or other substances. In a more profound feel, sobriety is an ongoing tool of restoration. The approach to sobriety addresses the muse cause of the substance abuse, how it took manipulate over the individual's existence, and the way they are able to get all over again heading inside the right course. Be it the addiction itself, a hidden intellectual condition that brought about it, or a coping mechanism to break out the stresses of lifestyles, sobriety addresses all of those. It focuses on liberating the person from the whole lot associated with their lousy addiction, from their beyond and into their destiny. The method also can even include highbrow fitness treatment and spiritual recovery along facet medical detox.

The blessings of sobriety range from a modern-day feel of well-being to progressed relationships. A few of the benefits of being sober encompass:

- Improved reminiscence (no thoughts fog and better crucial questioning and preference-making skills)
- Healthier pores and skin
- Improved everyday look

- Improved sleep
- Decreased danger of maximum cancers
- Better weight manipulate
- Healthier eating conduct
- Improved testosterone ranges
- Slower growing old
- Decreased irritation

While sobriety permits your inner organs to recover from alcohol-delivered about damage and, ultimately, enhance your physical health, it'll also permit you to see how ingesting changed into destructive your relationships with the people round you. Emotional balance is one of the maximum large benefits sobriety gives to the addict. Much like how ingesting in maximum instances impacts the significant fearful device—inflicting tension, tremors, and unique afflictions—abstinence initiates the restore of the stressful gadget to fitness inside the first few days.

Chapter 3: First Steps To Freedom

"You don't have to see the entire staircase. Just take the first step."
– Martin Luther King

Professional Help and Support

Alcoholism is the gateway to a myriad of troubles. The irony is, a number of the preliminary signs and symptoms are frequently brushed under the rug. Even even though alcoholism is maximum of the maximum huge public health troubles inside the United States, the trouble although fails to get preserve of top enough attention.

Many people find out it hard to govern their eating behavior in a few unspecified time inside the future of their lives. In the us, almost 15 million people had been recognized with AUD, with one in 10 youngsters living with a decide with AUD. Treatment of AUD does, in truth, paintings wonders. Regardless of methods intense the trouble, there's constantly want. A aggregate of highbrow fitness assist and medical remedy can loose an individual from the deadly keep close to of AUD.

An person have to right now are searching out expert assist inside the occasion that they experience any of the following symptoms:

- Memory issues
- Cold sweats
- Heart palpitations
- Yellowing of the pores and pores and pores and skin and eyes
- Swelling inside the legs
- Bruising effects
- Vomiting blood
- Dark urine and tarry searching feces
- A swollen belly

The above signs want immediately scientific intervention, as they may suggest advanced alcoholism. However, a proactive approach is a much better way to avoid the emergency room. Symptoms of alcoholism that signal the want for expert assist and assist encompass melancholy, restlessness, tension, nausea, sweating, insomnia, and irritability.

Individuals on the milder spectrum of the illness want to reap out to help groups that could help inside the initial tiers of AUD. Help is effects available online, which also lets in you to live anonymous if you desire. There are examined businesses similar to the Substance Abuse and Mental Help Services Administration, BetterHelp, and the National Institute on Alcohol Abuse and Alcoholism. You can start the gadget with a mobile phone name or through the use of filling out a web shape. Before you realise it, you're in a assist organisation in which you may start to share your troubles. Communication is important, so don't be afraid to allow it all out.

Support corporations permit individuals to talk to people who are or had been of their shoes and recognize what it looks as if to be afflicted by alcoholism. Group chats and professional intervention may additionally additionally moreover useful resource patients in lots of strategies. Counseling is a critical step on the street to restoration.

Expectations

When it consists of sobriety, expectations are frequently an extended manner from reality. This ebook doesn't offer an in a single day restore to 3 component as debilitating as alcohol addiction. It is, but, a guide for embarking on that adventure and tackling the hassle one step at a time. As cited earlier, the liver takes about an hour to metabolize one unit of alcohol. The greater you drink, the longer it takes for the liver to flush the alcohol from the body, not to mention the pollution it consists of that damage the liver and exceptional organs. Breaking the dependancy takes masses extra conviction than developing it.

To wreck the cycle, the primary 20-day rule applies. It's said that it takes 20 days, on common, to interrupt a addiction. With alcoholism, an man or woman can strive the 20-day rule to peer in which they stand. Don't circulate clean on your self in some unspecified time inside the future of that duration. Abstinence can assist in reducing tolerance to alcohol, making ingesting cautiously feasible. If you don't indulge your urge for those 20 days, strive for forty days. If now not whatever else, your body may also moreover need to apply the spoil.

Withdrawal signs start nearly right now, so anticipate the primary week to be tough. You also can experience the following signs and symptoms and signs and signs and symptoms within the ones weeks:

- Palpitations
- Breathlessness
- Dizziness
- Sleeplessness
- Nausea
- Diminished urge for food
- Paranoia

Once you overcome those barriers, you'll apprehend you're capable of surviving the journey in advance. Sometimes, signs and symptoms are extreme, and you could even need to be hospitalized. Medications like neuroleptics and benzodiazepines can be required collectively with a healthy eating plan. A bleak component-impact of sobriety is the danger of experiencing seizures, but proper treatment can lower the possibilities of these occurring. Withdrawal signs and symptoms and the accompanying treatment may additionally look like a large turnoff, however the initial hard stages of recuperation are critical for buying your lifestyles lower back. Keep an open mind and shift your interest to the present day-day "you" geared up at the alternative stop of the manner.

Mindset

For most people, becoming sober doesn't work on the number one attempt. The avenue to sobriety is a rollercoaster experience, and there might be times even as you'll revel in discouraged approximately ever getting sober. Sobriety itself is a difficult road, and there'll probable be episodes of relapse, binge consuming, and a go lower back of sobriety. The key to success is your strength of thoughts and your perseverance. The right mind-set is what's going to tug you through.

Understand that it's your lifestyles at stake. You didn't come this a long way to die an addict. Think approximately who you aspired to turn out to be whilst you were extra more youthful and what alcohol have become you into. You need to have finished better things had you now not fallen for something as insignificant as a horrific-tasting beverage in a glass. For your future and the sake of your circle of relatives, you want to reboot your lifestyles and start anew every time you relapse. Brighter days are searching in advance to you, so that you must regain your health.

Adapting a "increase mind-set" has helped people float ahead following setbacks. A increase thoughts-set is a practical method to conquering your dependancy. It encourages the notion which you'll benefit achievement to your efforts no matter how generally you've failed. Believing you're in whole control of your abilties will let you enhance and improvement. This is the actual key to fulfillment. With the right mind-set, humans will enhance their strength of mind and pull themselves thru.

With one of these tough adversary as alcoholism, it's k if you relapse. All you want to do is get lower back up and keep on the road to sobriety. Don't surrender until you get there— and you may. Persistence, strive, and hard paintings are crucial, but they aren't as vital as believing you're on top of things of your destiny.

Preparation

Addiction isn't this kind of subjects in lifestyles which you should rely on good fortune to help you conquer. Quitting an energetic dependancy takes a sturdy will, recognition, and preplanning so you can gain success. This doesn't even take into consideration the quantity of strive you want to live in restoration or maintain sobriety.

As any ideal self-help e book or teach will permit you to recognise, achievement comes from proper planning and practise. While it could appear that individuals who effectively reap their dreams do this thru achievement or that one unmarried destroy, we often brilliant see the forestall of the iceberg of the paintings that went into that precise success. The identical is actual for everyone who's attempting to interrupt freed from the chains of dependancy. It's smooth to be beaten by way of the use of the concept of getting sober. There are such loads of topics to bear in thoughts and moves to take that you could likely sense paralyzed.

The maximum great step in getting equipped yourself for the adventure in advance is growing an motion plan and committing to it. That willpower is available in elements. The first element is committing to this manner by manner of stepping throughout the starting line and quitting eating on day one. The second detail is an ongoing dedication to constantly propel yourself in the path of your goals and glide one step further a protracted manner from your alcohol use every day. Believe you may do it, and also you're midway there!

The endorsed motion plan for alcohol restoration has four elements: humility, motivation, perseverance in attempt, and the recuperation of love and cause for your existence. As the names of those 4 factors suggest, the movement plan has the entirety to do collectively collectively along with your highbrow fitness. Let's get into the records of the motion plan.

Set Short-term and Long-term Goals
Your plan has to have a time frame. We can get so caught up within the method of on the point of prevent consuming that we in no way step over that beginning line to do it. Procrastination can be a large trouble whilst dealing with something that could purpose you a few pain. This is why its so critical to set a specific time

body for beginning your journey and meeting your desires.

Use the following 3 inquiries to shape a framework for persevered movement:
1. What sports do I need to do to advantage my purpose, and in what time frame?
2. What property do I need?
3. Who can assist me reap my cause?

Take It One Step at a Time
Quitting alcoholism is tough, so starting up a five-year plan while you first start is illogical and farfetched. Keep it easy, and begin small. Reward your self for every step you accomplish, and replicate to your adventure. Be satisfied with your self for even going an afternoon without alcohol. If you gave in to the urge, recollect why you in all likelihood did that. There's continually a motive inside the again of the cause. Dissect the idea and troubleshoot the problem.

Record Your Progress

Alcohol use sickness isn't just about how a whole lot you drink but additionally how often, so you want to file both. If you relapse, document that too. As you improvement along the road to restoration, you'll have some element to reflect on and end up aware of the powerful results of abstinence. You'll locate that you're relapsing a whole lot much less than you have been a couple of months inside the past.

No depend how awful you can revel in at instances, don't allow the ill days inhabit your thoughts. Instead, interest on who you'll be a year from now. In the worst moments, inform yourself, "This too shall bypass," and do not forget in it.

Transitioning to sobriety is a gradual and ordinary method with many hurdles. Use a calendar to focus on days in which you had been a success. The visible markers will inspire you more than you don't forget.

Find Your Support Team

We live in a international wherein humans are continuously judged. You don't want to function for your anxiety through telling every body approximately your situation. Tell your near family and buddies that you're on the lookout for to forestall eating alcohol and supply an motive at the back of why. This way, you could percent your successes with them, and they'll understand why you've commenced declining drinks or journeys to the bar. Frequently reminding yourself and the human beings close to you why you need to prevent ingesting can assist hold you on path and may even inspire someone else to surrender or cut down collectively with you.

If you prefer to keep your adventure private and want ethical assist at any point in time, go online and sign on with a assist business enterprise that continues your identity anonymous. You can without hassle find a pal who is privy to what you're going through and engage with them approximately your issues. Communication enables loads at the same time as the individual you're speakme to is aware of what it's like.

Stay Dedicated

Recovery is all approximately motivation, so the motive that activate you inside the path of sobriety ought to be one which you could with out issues locate strength in. Recall this reason on every occasion you enjoy like having a drink. Reflect on who you've got were given been earlier than you started out ingesting or who you'll be while you save you. Persevere, and keep moving in advance.

Manage Triggers and Cravings

There are 3 primary facts about cravings that you want to deliver to mind on every occasion you've got were given a craving: cravings are time-limited, cravings don't ought to be happy, and ignoring a yearning received't harm you—in fact, pretty the alternative. An powerful way to address a craving is to divert your hobby as fast as you experience it. Take a touch stroll and distance your self from the state of affairs or human beings round you.

Abstaining from alcohol should likely look like the extremely good route to sobriety, but this could have some dire consequences. It may also pressure you to avoid pubs altogether or exit social sports wherein ingesting is the norm. Individuals with a strong dependancy may also even keep away from food that consists of a "sprint of alcohol." Regardless of the way harsh it may appear to your buddies and pals, abstinence have to take precedence due to the reality that's what's going to hold your life. You can continuously with politeness refuse invitations from human beings, and in case you understand them well sufficient, you may permit them to recognize you're in search of to get sober.

Replace Old Habits with New Ones
An motion plan like this may get you started on the road to restoration, however accomplishing the final intention of traditional sobriety doesn't appear fast. The movement plan lays the muse as a manner to get started. Regardless of ways insignificant your try may

moreover seem as compared to your addiction, the maximum critical detail is to start. The essence of sobriety comes all the way all the way down to changing your each day conduct. Replacing consuming with greater wholesome behavior is the manner you soar-start your restoration.

Alcohol addiction isn't an remoted conduct. It's continually a part of an horrific way of life. An horrific way of life isn't quite a great deal what you devour and drink. It includes terrible relationships, pressure, and precise varieties of hassle. If ingesting is the compensating mechanism in dealing with a disturbing courting, system, or state of affairs, you want to find a few other way to address this. We're surely now not suggesting that you abandon friends and circle of relatives due to the fact they stress you out. The secret's locating a manner to reduce that strain.

Focus on everything that alcohol is stopping you from doing and dedicate yourself to the obligations you've prolonged remove. Devote a while to paintings, family, and your nicely-being. Volunteering for network paintings may be very profitable, and you would in all likelihood meet humans going via the same transformation that you are, at least mentally. Love and excellent paintings are the high-quality benefits of life, so make certain you double-dip on the ones additives.

To replace your ordinary "Happy Hour," strive catching a few espresso with a chum. You'll discover more coffee drinkers than alcohol indulgers quite a whole lot anywhere. Spending happy hour with buddies and circle of relatives at domestic is a sincere higher concept. If this doesn't sound like a brilliant vibe for you, you could continually genuinely say no to alcohol, even at a pub with pals. You could have a non-alcoholic beer, in case you experience the flavor of beer, or a club soda. You ought to make the choice to live sober and still have a incredible time. It may moreover take some time to extend healthy behavior, but they'll massively beautify your lifestyles.

The Habit Chaining approach is quite powerful for folks with AUD. Introduced via using the Wall Street Journal bestselling writer, S.J Scott, the idea is that making small existence modifications for your behavior has quite an impact. "Build exercises round behavior that don't require strive" due to the truth "small wins construct momentum. They're easy to remember and entire," stated Scott in his 2014 ebook, Habit Stacking: ninety seven Small Life Changes That Take Five Minutes or Less. He proposed the precept of "addiction chaining," describing it as a way of grouping collectively small sports activities activities into everyday behaviors that in the end provide upward thrust to a new dependancy.

The "praise" is the subsequent step in solidifying a healthful addiction you've really created. When eating is changed with a modern pattern, the praise you apprehend in having a drink performs a critical role within the technique. Say the satisfied hour drink is a laugh not sincerely because of the booze buzz but additionally due to the reality you're putting out with pals and you may let out. You can nevertheless enjoy the equal camaraderie when you have a non-alcoholic drink as an opportunity. The new addiction you're growing may be a few component, and the praise, too, may be some thing you revel in. Dissect what offers you pleasure and recognition on what in reality feels profitable to you.

Remember, the essential aspect to developing any nicely dependancy is to be regular with it. Be determined to attain the reward you deserve and artwork inside the direction of it. Change is probably sluggish on the start, however the marginal profits will hold you in the long run. The energy of marginal income in sobriety performs a massive feature in recovery.

Achieving incremental dreams is all about the small information. If you're taking walks on sobriety, an incremental purpose have to embody searching after, say, your teeth. Since alcohol influences the fitness of your gums, you could lose your tooth pretty in advance in lifestyles. Alcohol moreover gives you horrible breath, so there's some other purpose to prevent. An adjunct gain of stopping eating is having easy breath. You're now thinking about superior oral hygiene in modern day. Good oral hygiene is now part of your existence and, earlier than you apprehend it, this will amplify to normal self-care. Why should you in fact limit problem about your frame to oral hygiene? You moreover want to have perfect pores and skin, this is related to ingesting a healthy food regimen, workout, strain-loose days, and further. This is the essence of a healthy manner of lifestyles—correct conduct.

Once you get into the healthful area, set a date to your calendar a 365 days from now. That's the day you assume proudly saying your sobriety. Focus on that date, and every time it receives difficult, take a look at subsequent yr's calendar and continue to be determined to achieve your quest. You apprehend you could do it.

Detox and Withdrawal

Alcohol affects the frame at a cellular diploma, which results in the sickness of the thoughts's neurochemicals. The neurochemicals emerge as imbalanced, which can be visible quick after a person has a drink. The withdrawal symptoms and signs and symptoms, too, are the stop cease result of this imbalance. The "withdrawal syndrome" takes place at the equal time as an man or woman with AUD abstains from consuming alcohol. Once your body has end up hooked on alcohol, the thoughts's major inhibitory chemical, GABA, and its maximum essential excitatory chemical, glutamate, grow to be dysfunctional. The thoughts's characteristic is primarily based totally carefully at the coordinated transmission of GABA and glutamate symptoms. These neurotransmitters are responsible for many talents. GABA plays a characteristic in how we enjoy anxiety, fear, and strain. And Glutamate is associated with reminiscence and analyzing. Impaired uptake of glutamate is associated with stroke, autism, a few kinds of highbrow disability, and ailments together with amyotrophic lateral sclerosis and Alzheimer's disorder.

Alcohol acts like a sedative, stimulating the frame to launch extra GABA. GABA blocks indicators and results in a slowdown in thoughts and worried device interest. This method alcohol hinders your cognition, influences your reminiscence and attentiveness, or even receives inside the manner of your potential to have interaction with people and situations.

The way alcohol influences the worried device consequences in acute withdrawal symptoms and symptoms that can be fatal. Binge drinkers, in particular, are prone to immoderate withdrawal symptoms and signs and symptoms, that is why heavy indulgers want to check with a doctor when they are looking to get sober. The first 14 days of abstinence can be the hardest because of some factor referred to as "the kick." If you can get through the primary 14 days, the entirety receives much less complex. Withdrawal signs normally have an impact on adult binge drinkers, but teenagers or greater youthful human beings with AUD also can revel in the consequences. The signs and signs and signs and symptoms are tough however can be treated. Therefore, expert supervision is vital.

The alcohol withdrawal way consists of the following 3 tiers:

Stage 1: The first six to 12 hours of alcohol detox. This is whilst you'll probably experience headache, nausea, stomach ache, and insomnia.

Stage 2: The subsequent 12 to 48 hours. This is on the equal time as signs can grow to be horrifying. Some people even experience seizures and hallucinations.

Stage three: The last forty eight to seventy hours, which might be the hardest. An person might also go through a racing heartbeat, excessive blood pressure, delirium tremens, sweating, fever, confusion, auditory hallucinations, and, doubtlessly, loss of life.

These withdrawal symptoms and signs and symptoms can deliver the mind's neurotransmitters into surprise due to the fact, as we've said, alcohol impacts the frame on a cell level, so the complete body is affected. This is exactly why you want to be beneath a expert's care at the same time as cleansing. Your age, weight, the depth of the dependancy, and awesome fitness issues want to be considered while growing your detox plan. Doctors and special healthcare specialists let you thru the detox and withdrawal ranges with the help of drug remedies like beta-blockers, anti-tension tablets, or different prescribed drugs.

Apart from all that, trying to detox at domestic is kind of generally vain while handling the kick. The urge to resume eating is probably strong, and lots of have a tendency to offer in. A boot camp or rehab facility is hundreds extra effective in supporting an man or woman to correctly and as it should be benefit sobriety. As cited earlier, you may experience setbacks, however seeking to stop consuming at domestic—if you have alcohol for your refrigerator, or you may effects stress to the store to get it—is a recipe for failure.

Chapter 4: The Approach

"It does now not depend how slowly you skip, best that you do no longer save you." — Confucius

Ironically, a volatile substance like alcohol stays criminal to shop for and use in maximum factors of the world. "Not sincerely all of us who liquids is an alcoholic," they are announcing, however commonly, absolutely everyone who liquids may be at risk of turning into one. The query is, why take that threat inside the first area? If there's nothing more valuable than lifestyles, why are we able to tempt fate as we do by means of way of the usage of risking harming ourselves? It most effective makes revel in that some detail that places your life at danger have to be avoided simply, but our collective societies foster alcoholism to a remarkable extent.

Treating AUD saves lives, and locating out the inspiration cause of the addiction is a revelation in the method. This e-book makes a speciality of four center elements involved in alcoholism: addiction, natural, mental, and social. Addressing the ones four middle elements will permit you to assemble a rock-strong foundation from which you could revel in a existence of sobriety for future years. You want to without a doubt embody each principle if you searching for prolonged-time period success. One of the number one overarching thoughts is completely committing to restoration in all areas of your existence. All of these elements paintings together. It's now not probable that you'll achieve lasting fulfillment with sobriety with out addressing they all.

Principle 1: Addiction

Alcoholism is a progressive illness, and prolonged alcohol abuse takes a toll in your health in lots of techniques. The in advance the trouble is detected and addressed, the higher to your fitness and your life. As stated earlier, the first step within the recovery way—after acknowledging you have were given were given a trouble—is detox. With the tough preliminary section of detox completed, you'll stumble upon the second one-hand challenges of abstinence. The whole technique to sobriety comes into question while triggers become strong. Sticking for your determination is the handiest manner via.

Managing triggers is what sobriety is all approximately. The question is, how do we strive this? A custom designed technique will help you control your triggers. There's generally a cause in the back of an urge, be it your frame's biological response to a stimulus or the outdoor surroundings or occasions that instigate the trigger. The following points will help you cut down the motives within the returned of your motivations.

Emotional episodes

Being an AUD sufferer is hard enough. It's a everyday battle. Gaining the braveness to face the reality that you have AUD and start running on enhancing your self are massive milestones. Some people also can need to save you communicating with pals and family for extended periods to stay robust in this approach. This can speedy take a toll on an individual's intellectual health, which may moreover already be compromised through a few years of alcohol abuse. There also can additionally come a point whilst feelings are overpowering and reason the urge the drink. When this takes place, it's important to recognize you may forget about the trigger and distract yourself from what's stressing you out.

Over-wondering
When you're in recovery, chemicals for your frame variety and make you enjoy you're on a roller-coaster of feelings and bodily effects. This may additionally additionally eventually lead you to over-wondering your choice to abstain, and you may even preserve in mind leaving behind your strive. This is all part of your recovery, so don't deliver in to your doubts and rationalizations. Feelings of hopelessness and negativity can from time to time rise up no matter your non-public issues. It's no longer you; it's a symptom of the restoration approach. Stay robust.

Trauma

Trauma is a large a part of human life, and it can be taken into consideration one of the most essential participants to highbrow health problems, which consist of depression, tension, and dependancy. According to the National Council for Behavioral Health, 70% of adults in the United States have skilled as a minimum one demanding occasion, this means that that 223 million human beings inside the US on my own have had trauma. Moreover, among dad and mom which is probably searching out remedy for mental health problems, ninety% have long long past via trauma.

Time doesn't constantly heal all wounds. It truely allows them to disappear into the historic past to make it tons less complicated with a purpose to undergo the day. The days in the long run end up less difficult, but the wound can also in no manner completely be healed, relying on the scenario. And that's ok. Some scars will in no manner in reality fade, and it's ordinary to be haunted through the usage of wonderful opinions. You don't want to get down on yourself for being emotionally caught up in the beyond every so often. Trauma and tragedy are a part of our lives.

When rehab and seclusion are part of your effort to get sober, traumas can every so often resurface and disappointed you. In truth, don't be amazed if a past trauma is reignited to a greater quantity in some unspecified time in the future of your days of recovery. This is why speaking to a counselor is an important a part of the approach. Triggers that you formerly attempted to deal with by means of eating will upward thrust up, so you need assist to create new conduct for handling unpleasant mind and recollections.

Your External Environment

There can be instances whilst even a advantageous environment will have you ever ever craving alcohol. It might be a meal you used to experience with a selected wine or possibly music which you always listened to with a drink for your hand. Smells, tastes, sounds, places, and even the climate also can purpose your urge, but you're on the street to restoration, so recognize the ones environmental triggers for what they're, and don't supply in.

If you do offer in, test what induced you and vow no longer to allow that take region over again. Even if it end up a entire-blown relapse, don't be discouraged. The cells in your body aren't under your command, and nearly absolutely everyone pursuing sobriety has relapsed at the least as quick as. A relapse is mostly a opportunity, so be organized for it. What subjects is that there's no cause it ought to prevent you from achieving your motive.

Principle 2: Biological

Your physical health performs a vital position in sobriety. Sleep, nutrients, and health are crucial elements in keeping and preserving a sober way of existence. Individuals affected by AUD are vulnerable to a deficiency of B-complicated vitamins which embody thiamine, folate or folic acid, and B12. There can also be a nutrients C deficiency. Meals wealthy in carbohydrates can assist restore your body to fitness. Pasta, bread, potatoes, carrots, beans, legumes, and lentils mixed with protein can help contrary the effects of alcoholism.

Principle three: Psychological

This precept makes a speciality of your intellectual fitness, which incorporates self-self warranty, spirituality, and emotional nicely-being. Sobriety is an extended journey, and a substantial a part of it consists of removing yourself from components of your preceding lifestyles. Boot camps and rehab centers are located a long way from towns just so citizens can get in touch with their proper self, free from distractions. Sobriety method recreating your way of life, which doesn't sincerely mean putting off alcohol from your bloodstream however furthermore purifying your headspace.

Meditating and focusing for your intellectual health play a essential role in healing. Beneficial mental factors will keep you ultimately. Developing a every day ordinary that continues you green and busy with meaningful paintings has helped many AUD patients. A awesome outlook on existence is what sobriety promotes, and an character beginning recuperation desires to make certain they include this idea to the fullest.

Principle four: Social

This principle focuses on assisting you select out, enhance, and amplify the right sorts of social relationships on your life inside the direction of restoration and past. Social constructs and relationships play the kind of large function in our normal existence, and they strongly resource or harm our opportunities of a a success recovery.

An AUD sufferer needs to find out a way to navigate each social setting in which ingesting is concerned. You want to study the way to say no to a suggestion of alcohol without feeling uncomfortable. It takes exercising, however you'll speedy have the ability to take part in quite a few social settings and stay sober. However, humans in restoration want to make sure their social environment permits their recuperation.

Addiction Focus
A Brief History of Addiction

Although this e-book is extensively talking dedicated to helping you for your adventure to freedom from alcohol addiction, we absolutely widely known the severa unique varieties of dependancy that have crippled generations and led humans to poverty, infection, and early loss of lifestyles. Addiction predates the recorded records of the Egyptian and Roman empires, but it wasn't till the advent of agriculture and farming that it became greater commonplace. Centuries later, a large amount of humans spherical the arena have come to be hooked on an entire lot of materials.

Approximately thirteen,000 years in the beyond, farmers grew addictive substances like marijuana, opium, and others. Because they will produce those materials in big quantities, dependancy witnessed a rise. Although plant-based totally addictive materials were highly smooth to deliver, in early times, their marketplace have emerge as constrained to particular regions due to the truth that wonderful plant life need to handiest develop on a specific shape of soil. In the 1800s, the area superior into the generation of chemistry and prescribed drugs. The advent of world trade allowed addictive materials alongside aspect amphetamine (1887), ecstasy (1912), PCP (1926), ketamine (1962), and distinct illicit capsules to be offered with out issue around the place

Substance abuse isn't new. What's alarming is that the charge of dependancy maintains to boom, and extra current, greater powerful, and additional risky materials are to be had. Some tablets can now prompt zombie-like behavior in humans, and a few tablets have drastic, long-time period effects on the frame. Addiction is a catch 22 state of affairs of modern-day society, and substance abuse is often part of the way of life of celebrities and particular famous figures, with alcoholism despite the fact that being taken into consideration one in every of its most famous office work.

The Addiction Cycle

The American Society of Addiction Medicine defines dependancy as a continual sickness that takes a toll at the abuser's reminiscence, motivations, and functionality to enjoy satisfaction and praise. Alcoholism is a contemporary disorder wherein feelings, behavior, and genetics may reason someone to move from some beverages a night time to binge consuming to the utilization of various addictive materials.

Addiction develops in stages. The cycle of dependancy is similar whether or now not the abused substance is alcohol or a bootleg drug. Just as with alcohol, the body develops tolerance to a drug, due to this greater and extra quantities are required to collect the same degree of effect. The aim is to interrupt this cycle. To achieve this, you want to first be privy to the tiers:

- Initial use
- Abuse
- Tolerance
- Dependence
- Addiction
- Relapse

Recovery endorses a backside-up technique to interrupt the cycle. Seeking treatment at a dedicated rehab facility reduces the possibilities of relapse, weans your frame off the addictive substance, reduces your dependence on alcohol or the illicit drug(s), and strengthens your solve, so your existence of abuse turns into records.

Fighting Addiction Is Hard
Individuals with AUD should spend years now not understanding they've a trouble. Even once they face it, stopping the addiction is a sizeable task. Nonetheless, the cycle can be interrupted,

and professional remedy has helped stored lives. Treatment in a rehab facility or with the assist of a expert is the final way to fulfillment. Alcohol recovery groups use protocols advanced through scientific research. The quantity of studies on alcoholism has finished wonders within the fight within the route of it.

There are a couple of types of treatment available for alcoholism. Cognitive-behavioral treatment has been verified to play a enormous function in supporting humans break out of the cycle of dependancy. Psychological issues stem from severa causes, with defective thinking patterns gambling a big characteristic. These patterns expand subconsciously underneath negative circumstances like a own family information of alcohol or drug abuse, adolescents forget about and abuse, despair, loneliness, social issues, a tough home environment even as the character is growing up, and peer/family pressure. Cognitive-behavioral remedy desires the wondering patterns that lead someone to are searching out secure haven in alcohol. It highlights the faults in an man or woman's perception of a given situation and lets in them to look subjects in any other case. This sort of treatment in the end rewires an individual's distorted patterns and unhelpful behavior, letting them correctly address tough situations instead of resorting to ingesting. Other kinds of adjunctive remedy for dependancy encompass peer assist agencies, medicine, and bodily remedy.

Setting a Quit Date
Sobriety focuses on looking ahead to dates an man or woman gadgets as benchmarks of their restoration. Each of those dates is celebrated, and that is a sturdy motivational component for an AUD victim. Clean dates or sobriety dates are milestones commemorating success and celebrating every different hazard at existence. These milestones may additionally want to embody the date a person quits ingesting, the date they join up in rehab, or the date they've long past a month with out a drink.

A sobriety date will permit an individual with AUD set a time frame and track their journey to be conscious their improvement and be an lousy lot a lot less in all likelihood to relapse. Keeping music of the days of sobriety is a effective a part of a a success rehab.

Although setting a give up date is appeared as a important element in undertaking healing, some have argued that placing a give up date can be unfavourable to the addict. Long-time 12-step critic Stanton Peele has argued that sobriety dates or easy dates instill feelings of disgrace and failure in folks who relapse. A change of mind-set is needed in this regard. To begin with, what distinct human beings say or anticipate doesn't take into account in phrases of questions of life and shortage of existence. A sobriety date ought to be taken into consideration a milestone to assist maintain you on target. If you relapse, you maintain going forward in conjunction with your restoration. As lengthy as you hold the mind-set of jogging on staying sober, you're a step in advance of who you've got been the day prior to this. It's a gradual and constant technique, and dates serve to document your improvement.

Identifying and Managing Triggers

Triggers fall below classes—outside and inner. Succumbing to a cause can drastically impact an person's recuperation, irrespective of its nature. Examples of a few triggers are:

- Depression
- Fear
- Grief
- Stress
- PTSD
- Abuse
- Feelings of unworthiness, disgrace, or guilt

Apart from the triggers referred to above, there can be precise triggers that make you liable to relapse, but if you have a sturdy treatment, you could resist. Managing triggers is all approximately self-reputation. The 2d you experience delivered approximately to inn in your antique methods of coping, question your self about what the stop result may be if you do this. Will alcohol treatment the trouble or make the reason lots a good deal less painful? It honestly acquired't. Will consuming assist you discover a technique on your pain? No, it received't. Does it damage you in case you don't react to the trigger with the beneficial aid of consuming? No, it doesn't. Identify what's triggering you and try and step out of your modern-day-day environment or distract your self in a healthful manner. Better but, talk to a counselor about your triggers so you're prepared to deal with them after they upward push up. A counselor can help you manage triggers, and ultimately, you received't reply to them anymore. Exercise, getting enough sleep, becoming a member of a assist group, meditation, and enjoyment activities also can assist you manage triggers more correctly. Triggers can be triumph over, so don't deliver in to them.

Recognizing Relapse Warning Signs

Relapse has been categorized into three factors: emotional, intellectual, and bodily. A relapse can display up on every occasion in a few unspecified time in the destiny of your recovery section, and the worst a part of it's far emotional in desire to bodily. It doesn't damage your frame to the degree it harms your motivation. The avenue to relapse begins prolonged earlier than you select up a drink. A relapse can sneak up on you, usually because you don't recognize the warning signs and symptoms.

Emotional Relapse
This is the maximum debilitating of the three factors and, sooner or later of this phase, you'll find out yourself struggling with the subsequent:

- Staying secluded or far from conditions that could reason you to drink
- Not attending your scheduled healing conferences and sports
- Failing to look after your self
- Poor ingesting and dozing behavior
- Mood swings
- Intolerance

- Paying greater interest to others to avoid your problems
- An everyday mind-set of not demanding about whatever
- Defensiveness
- Not accepting help

These signs need immediate attention. Journaling approximately your healing each day is a sensible and effective technique to averting a relapse. Deep respiratory, meditating, and developing greater positivity for your surroundings will help you snap out any dark thoughts and get you again on the right track.

Mental Relapse

When you turn a blind eye to an emotional relapse, possibilities are you'll fall prey to the second one aspect of relapse, that is the mental detail. Best described as a struggle inside oneself, a person present technique intellectual relapse takes on a twin personality: a person who desires to drink and a person who opposes the concept. An character also can input an almost trance-like united states of america, fantasizing approximately their break out from the determination they made. The intellectual relapse thing annoying situations the person to the center and will boom their vulnerability. The signs and signs and symptoms and signs and symptoms of highbrow relapse may furthermore include:

- Reverting to vintage behavior in desired
- Hanging out with pals who drink
- Reminiscing to others approximately past studies with alcohol or pills and boasting about it
- Lying
- Bargaining for why it's k to have a drink: "It's the vacations."
- Switching to other forms of substance abuse to alleviate the urge in a few manner
- Fantasizing approximately a relapse
- Trying to break out the restoration machine
- Missing out on scheduled conferences

Urges can final amongst 10 to half-hour, so stay positioned for at least that lengthy. Think about the results of what will show up in case you provide in. Think approximately all of the strength of will, suffering, and price you've continued to go back this a ways. Think about the priority you'd reason your family. Is one drink properly really well worth all that? Talk it over with a peer who is familiar with what you're going via. Be open approximately your thoughts and fears. Seek assist and undergo in mind: You've made it this a ways with out a drink, so that you can hold transferring ahead in your sobriety.

Physical Relapse
When someone doesn't take some time to widely known and address the symptoms of emotional and highbrow relapse, it doesn't take prolonged earlier than bodily relapse takes place. This includes the act of ingesting alcohol or the usage of one's preferred drug of desire.

Taking one drink may be considered a "lapse" or slip-up. Physical relapse is a move lower back to uncontrollable use. If this takes region, some people will hold to apply for months, at the same time as others recognize what they've completed and prevent loads quicker, returning their recognition to recovery.

After relapsing, precise steps can be taken to get yourself once more at the right song. Experts propose that those in recuperation do not forget situations in which they'll have the possibility to apply and rehearse what they'll do to save you a few different relapse.

Biological Focus
Food and water are the constructing blocks of existence. When it includes restoration, food performs a vital feature in restoring your frame's health. Some ingredients may also even contrary the debilitating consequences of alcoholism. Once you've launched into the road to restoration, unique modifications stand up interior your frame. Your frame starts offevolved offevolved offevolved healing finally of the detox level, and the alcohol-unfastened manner of existence requires some massive modifications in what you banquet on. Your immune device has been compromised by way

of using consuming alcohol, and which means that you want to consume a balanced healthy eating plan in order to supplement your frame with the right sort of nutrients.

In the preliminary days of detox, vomiting and feeling unwell could be the norm. You in all likelihood obtained't have plenty appetite for food, however don't be alarmed. This is a everyday part of the technique. A bad urge for food is exceptional transient. Nonetheless, you continue to need to eat a healthy eating regimen throughout the preliminary diploma as you look ahead on your appetite to head lower lower back. Long-time period AUD may also purpose deficiencies of nutrients on your body, and recovery focuses considerably on replenishing those deficiencies.

Nutrition

Nutrition is the inspiration of your physical fitness. Addiction can impact your physical body in lots of techniques counting on what you're addicted to, however aspect outcomes can include:

- Depletion of precise vital nutrients together with B vitamins (B1, B6, and folic acid)
- Damage to the liver and kidneys
- Imbalance of protein, electrolytes, fluids, and power
- Weight loss and malnutrition
- Mistaking emotions of starvation for cravings

Perhaps the most telling detail about nutrients is its impact for your highbrow nicely-being. Food plays a essential characteristic in assisting us to sense precise. According to the Mental Health Foundation, right nutritional selections are proper now related to higher tiers of mental properly-being. Eating a wholesome weight loss program is a clever way to construct a base from which recuperation can begin.

The 5 additives of a healthy weight loss plan have to encompass the following:

1. Keep Yourself Hydrated

Sufficient every day water consumption is usually vital, however this turns into particularly crucial at the same time as detoxing from alcohol dependancy. A cleansing of the body starts offevolved with assuring you're consuming hundreds of water. Ironically, notwithstanding the reality that alcohol is a beverage, it dehydrates the body. It's a diuretic, and as quickly as it enters your bloodstream, it flushes out vital nutrients thru the renal system. A diuretic motives the kidneys to flush fluids out of your body at a quicker price, and if you've been an AUD victim for long, you need to refill your frame's fluid ranges.

Once you're in detox, your body will start to flush out pollution, and vomiting and diarrhea are the most extreme detox effects. This is why eating hundreds of water is important.

2. Vegetables and Fruits
Studies have described a decrease in folate and vitamins A in people with extended alcohol abuse. Vegetables can allow an individual to experience complete without the greater power, and end end result are a more healthy opportunity to sugary cocktails that the

individual with AUD is aware of. Alcohol detox often induces cravings for sweets, and fruits will trick the thoughts into getting what it's annoying minus the alcohol. Experts receive as genuine with foods excessive in sugar stimulate the mind the identical manner alcohol does. A can of soda will do the same, however what's the factor of getting rid of one sort of chemical from your frame to update it with a few different? Eating some detail natural is the way to transport. Nutritionists recommend selecting complete give up bring about choice to fruit juices.

three. Protein
Alcohol assaults protein molecules particularly, so people stricken by AUD can increase a protein deficiency. Ethyl alcohol denatures protein, so it's critical that humans who've a statistics of alcoholism eat enough protein. Protein builds and continues muscle. A loss of protein could have dire results, which includes fatigue, decreased power, lack of muscle companies, and multiplied hazard of bone fractures. Poultry, fish, peas, beans, legumes,

nuts, and food regimen E-wealthy substances want to be covered into your eating regimen in a few unspecified time in the future of alcohol detox. Magnesium, iron, and zinc degrees need to be checked as well.

four. Whole Grains
Carbohydrate deficiency is not unusual in people with AUD. Alcohol helps the esterification of carbohydrates, which could result in hypoglycemia. Carbs are a extremely good deliver of fiber and energy, which the AUD sufferer often doesn't eat enough of. Sobriety is all approximately a easy frame, due to this eating wholesome, unrefined meals. Make high-quality your carbs are nutritionally complete in preference to processed grains. Whole grains like quinoa, brown bread, and oats are rich in vitamins B and a tremendous deliver of carbohydrates.

five. Savory Soups
Sobriety without a doubt doesn't recommend that while you prevent consuming alcohol you have got permission to eat a few element you

need. Detoxing your body is all approximately staying match, energetic, and refraining from consuming dangerous materials. Alcohol is poisonous for your frame, so because you've decided to save you ingesting to beautify your health, you want to keep away from lousy, processed meals.

Soups are a great manner to transport while cleansing, specially if you're managing nausea, indigestion, and vomiting. Be effective the soups are organized from scratch and no longer using a synthetic factors.

A balanced weight loss program will maintain your body through the recuperation segment and facilitate its healing from alcoholism. Keep in mind that cleaning from alcohol is hard in your body, so you need to address it nicely in the direction of the method. Detoxing will frequently make you lose your urge for meals and shed kilos, so that you want to top off out of area vitamins.

Fitness and Exercise

The word "fitness" strikes fear into the hearts and minds of many people. Our aware and unconscious minds still hold in mind those hard bodily training education at university. As adults, we're expected to keep on a physically active life-style on our very own. Thanks to an business enterprise built round making human beings experience terrible about their look, we've out of area the information of what it way to be healthful.

For those in restoration, we need to modify this definition. Fitness may be a in reality effective pressure in every preserving and playing sobriety. It may be tempting to handiest take into account health as something you do to try and lose a few pounds or get the ones six-% abs. However, fitness need to be notion of no longer as definitely a way of undertaking a few bodily benefit however as some issue that nourishes your entire being.

Ground-breaking discoveries approximately the useful consequences of exercising and fitness have taken the detox system to an entire exclusive diploma of fulfillment. Engaging in exercising modifies the mind's pathways and rewires the reward tool, that can flip topics spherical for the AUD victim. Exercising releases endorphins, the feel-appropriate chemical materials within the body, so that you have a feel of delight following a amazing exercising. Exercise can also increase your power degree and beautify sleep extraordinary..

Withdrawing from alcohol isn't most effective a conflict that takes vicinity in a single's thoughts however moreover inside the bodily body. Vomiting and diarrhea cause a person to revel in tired and coffee on strength, so start gradual in the end of your restoration with quick walks outdoors. As the instances bypass, the person want to put in force a exercising routine at a gym or specific setting. Focusing on the body makes it lots less difficult to address the urge to drink.

Sleep

Pulling your self via a huge contamination like alcoholism isn't quite a good deal a change of way of lifestyles but a exchange of the body as properly. You'll experience and notice the distinction in yourself as you get more healthy, due to this you've transitioned right into a cutting-edge and advanced you. Although this could no longer be as obvious in your look, the transition has a great impact from a highbrow attitude.

In this regard, sleep performs a enormous function. Rest heals the frame. When it involves the emotional strain of withdrawal, sleep is important. From stopping dementia to inhibiting the development of diabetes, precise enough, actual-great sleep is crucial.

The signs and symptoms and signs of withdrawal from alcohol have an effect on sleep styles extensively. During the number one week of detox, humans often experience insomnia. Individuals also can doze off without issues but awaken within the midnight feeling agitated. Some may want to probable find out it difficult to sleep and can document their sleep isn't restorative. Disrupted sleep styles are what motive a majority of AUD patients to relapse.

Alcohol works its magic thru using setting an person right right into a short, deep country of close eye. This is precisely why many people with melancholy or tension hotel to alcohol. Most withdrawal symptoms clear up through the years, but sleep problems take longer to restore. The Substance Abuse and Mental Health Services Administration (SAMHSA) said that 25% to 72% of human beings with alcohol use sickness document sleep issues. In recuperation, cognitive behavioral therapy for insomnia (CBT-I) may be useful to an individual having issue slumbering. Other remedy options consist of drugs, aromatherapy, non secular healing, and additional.

Fueling Your Body's Capacity to Heal

A aggregate of diet, exercising, sleep, and mindfulness will art work wonders in assuring you live at the course of sobriety. Nonetheless, breaking loose from AUD requires professional assist that includes remedy and, frequently, medicine. A rehab facility continues music of all additives of your physical properly-being, out of your fitness records to the modern-day country of your body. Blood paintings and examinations will show any regions of scenario, so any critical movement is taken in a nicely timed manner. Supplements and an incredible food regimen can be all that's wished for some individuals, even as others may additionally need greater in depth remedy if alcohol has damaged their important organs.

The element is, surely absolutely everyone is specific, and no longer each AUD sufferer may additionally have the identical signs and symptoms and symptoms and symptoms and symptoms and signs. A custom designed approach is wanted to gas the frame to maximize its restoration capability. Connecting with a dietician is a proactive technique in growing a greater wholesome lifestyle even as cleansing and afterward. A diet plan may be designed to satisfy your desires. Alternatively, are in search of a peer business enterprise that's involved in vitamins schooling to help you create a diet plan.

A beginner in recovery may additionally moreover moreover sometimes experience sick really on the sight of meals. Small and wholesome food consumed 4 or five instances a day can assist construct your tolerance for and interest in consuming. Under a expert's care, you'll locate approaches to address the ones thing consequences of healing. What need to take priority is making sure your weight loss program includes more than a few healthful elements and plenty of water.

Chapter 5: Psychological Focus

Mastering Your Mental Health

There's a dishonest in maximum cultures to avoid discussing our intellectual fitness with others, and consequently it's turn out to be a taboo trouble. We keep things in and mask our actual feelings, which creates pressure over the years. These withheld feelings and thoughts can impair our selection-making capabilities. As someone in recovery, growing your potential to make accurate alternatives is crucial.

If you stumble upon a capability relapse motive while preserving onto bottled-up feelings, you won't be capable of assume virtually or rationally. Being on top of factors of your thoughts, feelings, and ideals can be a unique concept. Your highbrow health calls for ongoing interest and care in the course of your lifestyles. It protects and gives the manipulate you want, specifically in recuperation on the equal time because the reason is prolonged-term sobriety.

Addiction can also moreover have taken manage of your lifestyles without you being conscious it have emerge as taking vicinity, but in case you've made it this some distance analyzing this e-book, you presently understand that addiction is curable. With the strength of your thoughts, you could triumph over it. The actual statistics is, you don't ought to do any of this on my own. Depression, anxiety, and different highbrow health issues are a part of every person's life, but in sufferers with AUD, the ones are more common. From outpatient help to inpatient remedy, you can reap expert assist while you're faced with psychological issues while you're going thru withdrawal.

A guaranteed hack to preserve a wholesome mind-set is to recognize you're enhancing your life each day you don't drink. Many of your issues will surrender, and every passing day brings you closer to your future. Substance abuse is curable, and also you're already to your way to recuperation. What changed into the use of you to alcoholism is not in fee. The worst is inside the lower lower back of you, and also you're properly along your adventure even as you make a decision to get sober. Don't permit a illness define your existence.

Living Intentionally
For a few, "dwelling deliberately" approach having a clean intention for each motion. In alcohol healing, residing intentionally manner having a proactive approach wherein the primary motive is to improve your health mentally, emotionally, and bodily. Looking after the body requires hobby to bodily goals like meals, water, and sleep. A huge part of intentional living is the employer perception within the price of living within the present 2nd and setting desires. It moreover promotes kindness, empathy, and being grateful for the blessings in our existence.

Living deliberately is specially beneficial in recovery because of the truth it is able to help save you an man or woman from having a relapse. Setting small goals for every day—in particular if it's a bad day—facilitates save you human beings from bouncing all over again into their antique behavior.

For example, bear in mind this situation: Lisa is 16, and he or she or he had a bad day at university. She became made amusing of, and the person she likes asked some different woman out. The instructor scolded her for now not paying interest, and she or he felt embarrassed. When she were given domestic, she changed into her pajamas and binge-watched Friends episodes till she dozed off. The following day, Lisa have been given up and went to highschool feeling plenty better. On the alternative hand, Bill is forty eight, and he was picked on at artwork. The manager regarded to find fault with the whole thing he did. He had a heated argument with the manager and left his project early to try to switch off his mind, virtually as Lisa did while she watched all of the ones episodes of Friends. Since Bill has AUD, he went immediately to the liquor store and purchased six-packs of beer. He went home and drank until he surpassed out.

If Bill had lived deliberately that day, he wouldn't have resorted to ingesting. Every motion need to have a easy motive of living with motive. Binge eating has no motive in any respect, and that's wherein Bill would in all likelihood have drawn the road had he lived deliberately. He didn't set small dreams for his day—like staying on the place of job till his normal time to leave, going domestic and beginning up about his day to his spouse, having dinner along with his own family, after which dozing off to evoke with a clean head for the following day at art work.

Living intentionally we may want to humans take steps a very good way to advantage their intellectual health and contribute to their experience of contentment. It diminishes behaviors that harm the body and might help do away with procrastination and lousy questioning styles.

Prioritize Wellness and Self-care
Self-care is one of the maximum critical elements of healing. Active alcohol use may

additionally moreover have left you neglecting yourself and your number one dreams. As an alcoholic, you might have spent days in mattress. Poor hygiene, an unbalanced healthy eating plan, and a deteriorating social lifestyles are all repercussions of self-neglect. In recovery, you do the alternative. The cardinal precept of recuperation is to prioritize yourself and address your needs regardless of what. Some may want to probably assume this sounds egocentric, but whilst it's AUD we're speaking approximately, self-love is critical.

Small acts of self-care like taking an extended heat shower, shopping for your self some factor you want, meditation, and good enough sleep assist alleviate pressure and make your healing much less complex. The overlook your frame persisted on the same time as you were underneath the have an impact on of alcohol desires to be reversed. While medicinal drugs and detox deal with you from the inner, acts of kindness to your self and mindfulness will cope with you from the outdoor. Only you can pull your self via, so supply yourself lots of love and disturbing.

Positive Mindset
The idea of getting a awesome thoughts-set in recuperation is often misconstrued. Being terrific doesn't mean you need to placed on a colourful face even at the same time as you feel like lack of life at the internal. A notable mind-set has to do collectively along with your idea system. It approach typically focusing on the effective aspect of factors in desire to the terrible. Being an AUD sufferer is a grim state of affairs, but there's a treatment, so recognition at the remedy. Asking for help is a extremely good gesture, on the equal time as retaining your dependancy bottled inner or neglecting it acquired't help you.

A effective mind-set will make the restoration phase loads smoother. Believing in yourself and know-how you deserve every little little bit of love and interest to procure—from yourself or others—is what positivity is about. Even in case you relapse, live nice and realise it's all part of the game. When the going gets tough, believe that you'll pop out more potent. Believe in yourself, and hold going.

Affirmations

Never underestimate the electricity of phrases. Hurtful terms spoken to us can stay with us for all time. Words have delivered approximately revolutions and feature destroyed entire groups. When in recuperation, the strength of phrases intensifies. Affirmations are an extension of the nice mindset we said earlier. Reciting or studying affirmations is a workout that destroys discouragement and negativity.

Words we inform our self often have a more massive impact than what someone else tells us. In healing, awful mind and emotions are an impediment. The technological knowledge of affirmations endorses the identical ideology. A test posted in the mag Social Cognitive and Affective Neuroscience used MRI to show the effect of terms at the reward facilities in the thoughts. Repeating awesome phrases like, "I deserve a higher existence" or "One step at a time" will assist spark off the thoughts's praise centers, augmenting the incentive an person in recovery desires.

Other wonderful phrases or affirmations which can be empowering encompass:

- "I love myself."
- "I'm sufficient to make myself glad."
- "Progress doesn't suggest I want to be perfect."
- "I'll never give up."
- "I get hold of as true with I can do that.

Managing Stress
Stress performs a splendid role in relapse, and that's exactly why managing strain takes pinnacle precedence in rehab. Stress isn't avoidable but it's potential. From minor problems like being late for university to extra essential troubles like a awful dating, strain can take a toll to your lifestyles even whilst you're sober. The following strategies will assist you manage strain better:

- Meditation: Meditation permits you to witness your mind and be capable of see past the traumatic state of affairs to the larger image. It offers you a hen's eye view and creates distance between you and your hassle, permitting you to view it more honestly. It may additionally furthermore even assist you to discover a way to what's inflicting you stress.

- Let it out: Be it crying or clearly organising up about your problems with a expert or a peer, talking out your feelings helps you to way the strain and reflect onconsideration on a situation from a unique mindset. It lets in you to expect out of the field and apprehend that something is stressing you out will bypass, and you'll pull through.

- Socialize: Stepping from your conventional surroundings for some time and catching up with buddies and own family can increase your mindset and be a superb de-stressor. You'll gain insight into their lives and conditions and realize you're now not the only one going through disturbing activities. A little diversion and slight-hearted laughter advantages pretty a great deal absolutely everyone. Just make sure your liquids aren't part of your socializing.

Willpower
Without strength of thoughts, sobriety is pretty masses an illusion. Although power of mind by myself can't assist you obtain sobriety, it performs a important position. Scientific studies define energy of thoughts as:

- The potential to restrain oneself from carrying out terrible actions
- The capability to manipulate one's urges
- The determination to keep one self through hard patches in life
- Self-problem
- The functionality to stay steadfast toward temptations to achieve extra rewards

In recuperation, power of will is vital to each gain and sustain the sobriety you're striving to accumulate. An character with AUD will face infinite temptations to relapse. Willpower is needed, and if it's robust enough, not anything can save you you from accomplishing your goals.

Avoiding Temptation

When you're inside the initial phases of restoration, you need to lower pressure, drama, temptations, and every element that could cause you into relapsing. Going out along with your consuming friends or frequenting consuming locations and eateries that feature alcohol is a no-no for the abstainer. Do your self a prefer and remove whatever for your life as a manner to make it greater difficult if you want to abstain. Explore new places to satisfy buddies, eat, and feature fun in which alcohol isn't to be had. You'll brief find out there are numerous greater methods of playing yourself than clearly getting underneath the have an impact on of alcohol.

This can be the right opportunity to boom your horizons and find out new cultures, cuisines, and enjoyment that don't encompass eating. Yes, there are locations in the international in which alcohol isn't a part of a few component.

Meeting new human beings and mastering greater about their way of lifestyles and norms will help you benefit a larger mind-set on lifestyles, permitting you to understand how restricting a lifestyles that's fueled through alcohol can be.

Journaling

Journaling about your recuperation is a terrific manner to reflect to your achievements. Don't fear if you haven't finished any of the responsibilities you placed for your self on a specific day. You can nonetheless write down your mind and emotions, and also you'll see the distinction it makes. Psychologists agree with journaling brings clarity to the thoughts and encourages attention of your personal mind and motivations. In the technique of writing, you will possibly experience like breaking down and crying, that is a step in the direction of emotional recovery. You may additionally even provide you with a way to a few component you're careworn approximately or have been searching for to decide out. This will display your real internal information and assist you to rate your self all the more.

Journaling is a personal document that you could use to track your recovery as well as something to mirror on. It's an act of self-care that permits you reputation to your abilties, your flaws, and the answers available. It's also an act of self-mastery, and thinking about that recuperation has lots to do with reading your electricity of mind, journaling plays a important position.

Chapter 6: Social Focus

We stay in an age enthusiastic about socializing and being well-known. Loners are often appeared upon as unusual, dysfunctional creatures who satisfaction in their lifestyles of solitude. Although keeping to oneself is a super idea at instances, it's no longer a healthful scenario in the long run. Family bonds and pals are what lifestyles is prepared. Just as social settings can lead you down the route to alcoholism, the proper form of social putting will will will let you recover from it, too.

Family and pals deliver meaning to life. They make life genuinely really worth stopping for, but that absolutely doesn't recommend you want to undermine your experience of self esteem to assist or please a few one-of-a-kind. It's proper which you're whole and sufficient on your own happiness, however this doesn't offer the same delight you enjoy whilst you may have an extraordinary time your lifestyles with those you like. Humans are constructed to be social creatures, so we should cope with our social dreams. Nonetheless, your social circle can, at times, intrude collectively together together with your quest for sobriety. Let's discover this in element.

Family and Friends

Speaking, questioning, and great journaling may be on your manipulate—and those can clearly make a contribution considerably for your restoration—however what about the elements for your lifestyles that you haven't any control over? Friends, family, and relationships are a part of existence—and probable what makes existence sense whole—but what if those closest to us sabotage our recuperation?

Alcoholism is everywhere, and chances are, you aren't the most effective one struggling with the ailment—regardless of the truth which you is probably one of just a few looking for sobriety. The sad reality is that maximum AUD sufferers don't want to face their hassle and received't are looking for assist. An character with AUD typically has a own family records in which at least an additional person has the identical hassle.

At instances, there may be humans spherical you who don't guide your sobriety or will actively attempt to sabotage it. They can be a member of your close to own family or a chum round the corner. In conditions in that you experience like someone is interfering together along with your efforts to get sober, you can try the following:

-   Avoid putting out with that individual in the event that they encourage you to percentage a drink with them.
-   Learn to mention no. Politely excuse your self from conditions that may cause a relapse.
-   Come up with an exit plan to transport away on the same time as a state of affairs receives too "drunk" spherical you.
-   Don't pay attention to those who are skeptical approximately your capacity to get sober.

- Be affected character with folks that discover the modern day you to be a stranger. It will take time for the human beings round you to adapt to your calmer man or woman.

Professional Relationships

In the expert global, you'll need to stand comparable conditions. Unfortunately, professional environments are some of the maximum hard for folks who are looking to recover from an dependancy or inside the intervening time are sober. Whether you're in university or have a career, your dependancy has sincerely made an effect on in which you are nowadays. How you technique and cope with your professional relationships can assist or forestall your future fulfillment.

There's no person-length-suits-all technique even as dealing with relationships at college and artwork. You need to learn how to check the room and recognize your contemporary-day situation. At a few factor, you'll ought to determine if and how you want communicate approximately your dependancy in a professional putting. You'll want a backup plan, and also you additionally want to learn how to distance yourself from toxic coworkers or classmates.

You might also additionally want to realize on the same time as speakme to a person higher up is crucial and how to tell in case you need to begin looking for a current technique. Thinking via a whole lot of these conditions can experience overwhelming. However, in case you're organized and characteristic belief via maximum capability situations, you could thoroughly navigate the expert international at the same time as fending off troubles regarding recuperation and sobriety.

For example, your boss might also be given as real with that ingesting is an important social interest and, as an expert discern, they might not attain your recovery and try to intimidate you into having a drink. The superb way to deal with conditions like this is to say no in a well mannered way. You may additionally must attend a agency dinner, and you'll be asked to make a toast. You can however make a toast and fake to drink without sincerely doing so, thereby maintaining your professional relationship whilst not sabotaging your sobriety.

There's normally a steady area in the middle someplace, and all you want to do is find out your manner to it. Opening as an awful lot as art work colleagues approximately your struggles isn't expert. Staying diplomatic but business enterprise to your convictions is the manner to head. Don't make a element of the way you aren't eating but clearly hold on with what you're there for. This is the top notch manner to painting a disciplined picture and maintain expert relationships sturdy.

Seek Support from Safe People

Knowing who "safe humans" are is top in healing. It's exquisite to surround your self with folks that received't select out or criticize you. The steady humans in your existence could be your friends and own family, or it may be a counselor if you revel in you want a piece greater assist than your private circle of guide can provide you.

Find help and are looking for comfort in folks that recognize a manner to pay attention empathetically with out feeling they need to say what they suppose you have to do. Seek consolation in the human beings whom to have the potential to pay hobby with compassion and feature examined kindness for the plight of others. Empathic listening abilties might also additionally seem clean to find out among friends and own family, but this isn't always the case. Most people find it tough no longer to allow preconceived notions or biases create judgments approximately those who are in search of to get over substance abuse. Most human beings may rather communicate about what's thrilling or beneficial for them. To be capable of interest definitely on each other individual's existence while there's no longer something in it for you is a virtually selfless act and an extended way more difficult to grasp than primary listening capabilities. It requires you to stroll a mile within the person's shoes with the resource of manner of experiencing their emotions. You get to experience their happiness, disappointment, ache, pleasure, misery, and the demanding situations they face almost as even though it have become your journey. You'll often find out that those who've suffered from dependancy are the suitable to speak to.

It will take time to create your guide tool due to the truth constructing be given as true with takes time. So, take some time to construct your help group, and make certain you select folks that'll unselfishly resource you and contact you out whilst needed.

Sobriety Success
"Somebody once asked me how I outline sobriety, and my response grow to be 'liberation from dependence'." — Leslie Jamison

It's the moment you've lengthy been expecting, and also you've marked this due to the fact the day of your rebirth. It's the start of a brand new existence, new recollections, and a ultra-modern you. You've earned the right to rejoice it, skip smooth on your self, and do the property you constantly favored to do. Reaching success in sobriety manner you're not a slave to alcohol. You've taken your power decrease lower back, and your thoughts and frame are in the long run underneath your command in region of your dependancy controlling you.

Now that you've finally walked the lengthy, winding avenue to the exit, , first-hand, how beautiful a sober life is. You see how masses much less complicated your lifestyles has emerge as. You've visible buddies coming returned into your lifestyles, you're getting invited to occasions and social gatherings, and also you're residing lifestyles to the fullest. You no longer feel scared that alcohol will regain a keep on you, even in a state of affairs in which drinks are being pressed on you. You revel in comfortable selecting an alcohol-loose beverage.

Recognize that there's no longer some factor incorrect with needing to be by myself once in a while, and you shouldn't enjoy responsible for giving yourself a treat every every now and then, every. It doesn't make you selfish to popularity on your self for a piece of time every day. You want that point to reorient your mind and stay strong for your recuperation.

People often inquire from me whether or no longer sobriety may be lengthy-time period. People need to apprehend if they might ever cross decrease returned to the lifestyles they as soon as had or have a drink every occasionally. To this query specifically, I say this: "No, you can't flow returned to that life, and nor should you need to. You left that existence especially as it was dangerous, detrimental, and affected you negatively in limitless techniques."

Sobriety is an prolonged-time period desire. Here are some hints to help at the side of your adventure:

- Make time for exercising. While many human beings forget about this, you need this time. Find sports that you love or normally preferred to try.
- Give your self a spa day, and do it to the max.
- Keep a magazine to mirror on the manner you experience.
- Stay in contact together with your emotional and physical wishes.
- Keep your treatment wishes organized (using a calendar or special planning device) to make certain you're taking medicinal pills or attend instructions or appointments as a manner to maintain you sturdy and targeted.
- Celebrate milestones with the useful resource of treating your self to some component first rate. It normally feels worthwhile to preserve up a hint cash and deliver our self a few element unique.
- Take time far from your devices because they might reason sleep troubles and distract you from your dreams.
- Learn the way to admire the notable outside. One of the excellent stress relievers is

to spend time in Nature. The clean air and the wonders of the Earth can revive your spirits. You don't need to spend a whole lot of time in Nature to start seeing the outcomes. Any place in Nature that you like will do. If you live in an city vicinity, finding a park or tending to houseplants or a community garden may be appropriate options. Even honestly half of of an hour in keeping with day spent in the herbal global could make you feel better, and you may combine your outdoor time with bodily hobby for added benefits.

- Find films or podcasts on addiction and healing so that you can examine from the studies and demanding conditions of others and notice how they have been in a function to triumph over even the most dire situations.

Now that you're for your way to improving from this disorder don't lose track of the intellectual growth and place you've received. Foster it with more understanding by way of the use of manner of studying books on alcohol addiction. Reading approximately what you've been via will remind you of your energy and perseverance each time you underestimate your functionality. Stay in contact with people for your beneficial resource agencies, and volunteer to paintings to assist others stricken by dependancy. There's now not some element extra lovely than sizable paintings, and what better way to rejoice your fulfillment than thru helping dad and mom that are going thru what you've skilled. This is what's going to maintain your recuperation for a lifetime.

The Challenge
With plenty outside stress in current society to be their first-rate selves, tens of tens of thousands and thousands of human beings international struggle to hold their intellectual health and professional or personal well-being. Many emotionally and physical risky behaviors—which include overworking and excessive self-sacrifice—are glorified by using using society. As people are pushed to do their notable artwork and make room for a personal and social life, they may emerge as ate up by

using anxiety and concerns that restrict their improvement.

The statistics on pressure, tension, and melancholy depict a grim picture. As the most popular highbrow fitness problem in the United States, constant with the Anxiety and Depression Association of America, tension impacts over forty million American adults, representing over 18 percentage of the populace. Globally, nearly 3 hundred million people have tension. People who have tension have a tendency to have extra strain levels, and 50 percentage of these diagnosed with anxiety will also be identified with despair. Depression prices also are startlingly excessive, with just underneath seven percentage of the population experiencing essential despair at any given time and every other percentage experiencing continual depressive sickness, additionally known as dysthymia or chronic melancholy.

Even if you don't have a clinically identified trouble, along with despair or tension, you likely have a few degree of stress that makes it extra hard to feature as you need to. The Global Organization for Stress says that seventy five percentage of people are fairly compelled, and nearly all people enjoy strain ultimately of their lives because of a myriad of contributing elements. With a lot mental sickness, it's no marvel that some humans expect they'll by no means get higher, but this grim photo doesn't ought to be your fact.

While highbrow fitness situations have the electricity to wreck and debilitate humans— paralyzing them and making it difficult to have preference for the destiny— there are examined techniques all people can use to beautify their intellectual fitness and allow greater possibility for personal improvement. You do not want to allow your stress, anxiety, or despair maintain you over again anymore.

The method to dealing with your intellectual health isn't easy or short, however it is powerful. With attempt and careful interest to a multi-faceted plan, you can make dramatic improvements on your broken intellectual health and start making an investment more power into matters that make you the most gratified. There are severa steps you need to study for the tremendous consequences. When you check those steps, you can have extended mental readability, emotional freedom, and self guarantee. Curing your highbrow health issues should require you to stand the whole lot that scares you and to confess uncomfortable truths. Still, you'll be a ways better off at the same time as you are looking for help than the nearly 25 million Americans who've untreated intellectual fitness conditions. You may not need the equal degree of care as humans with greater intense situations, but you do want assist because dwelling with any degree of strain, anxiety, or depression is living with more ache than you want to have.

Treating a intellectual infection can seem intimidating to many humans, but there are various effective strategies, and there are strategies to cope with, if not treatment, any highbrow health situation you may have. With such a lot of adults and children not currently being treated for his or her intellectual health issues, it's no wonder that intellectual health statistics live so everyday. Still, with elevated reputation and the greater availability of intellectual health belongings, the analysis for those who've highbrow contamination maintains to enhance. Alongside this, as those problems turn out to be extra extensively stated and noted, the stigmas associated with them are beginning to burn up, which receives rid of a number of the disgrace connected to intellectual contamination, which pleasant exacerbates it. Accordingly, via committing bravely to remedy and commencing yourself to elevated know-how of intellectual contamination, you create resilience in competition to intellectual contamination and become more proactive in the treatment of these debilitating situations.

For those of you with any of these issues, you can not eliminate remedy. Mental ailment of any type makes it more tough to enjoy pleasure and, within the worst times, it may deprive you of your capacity to function. More than that, your intellectual fitness also can effect your bodily health. For instance, studies has demonstrated that strain will increase the risk of a person demise from most cancers through 32 percent. The Canadian Mental Health Association says that human beings with terrible highbrow health are greater vulnerable to having continual physical problems.

A have a look at from Johns Hopkins University observed that patients with a own family data of heart disease had been greater wholesome after they engaged in extraordinary questioning. Among the contributors of the test, people who had a tremendous outlook were thirteen percent a good deal less probable to enjoy a cardiac event. Additionally, they determined that, generally, humans who have better outlooks stay longer.

The Solution

Recovery is a technique that isn't usually linear, however this ebook will lay out the primary steps to help get you at the right song. The first step within the method is all approximately schooling. Before you could do something else, you want to understand the beast you're looking for to slaughter and the sword you'll use to slay it. You'll discover how the brain works and the way troubles with its wiring can bring about intellectual ailment. You'll moreover examine the way you may rewire your cognitive methods to sell progressed mental fitness.

In the second step of the gadget, you'll preserve your academic adventure and benefit a better information of what tension, pressure, and depression are and the way they effect the manner you characteristic. You'll begin to recognize a way to cope with every of these troubles using crucial coping system.

Once you've positioned out about each scenario, you'll be brought to one of the most effective intellectual system for superior mental fitness: Cognitive Behavioral Therapy (CBT). You'll find out what CBT is and the manner to apply it to deal with your intellectual ailments.

Once you recognize the founding ideas of those conditions and the fundamentals of CBT, you'll discover ways to manage your times every day by means of manner of the usage of overcoming roadblocks and reviving your revel in of self by using manner of manner of transferring your mindset as you start to think in new techniques. You'll start to care for every your body and your thoughts in life-converting strategies. All of these steps will reason mental readability and intellectual liberation.

With all this in thoughts, it's clean that a person's highbrow fitness affects each part of their lifestyles, and with out addressing your intellectual disease, you'll in no way have the peace of thoughts you crave. Each day you do now not some element approximately your highbrow fitness is every other day you deprive your self of health and happiness. Your highbrow fitness need to be your precedence, because of the fact you can't surely characteristic as a member of society if you're prohibited from doing all the belongings you need the maximum.

If you experience like you're losing sight of yourself and your goals due to your pressure, tension, or despair, it's time to make a exchange. It's okay to be concerned approximately the modifications you could want to make to feel healthier, however do not forget that being uncomfortable and uncertain is vital due to the fact they constitute change. If you do now not trade, you can in no manner enjoy higher than you do now. Maybe you have got determined out to live collectively along with your pain and worry, however it is time to discover ways to stay without the ones poor coping mechanisms because they prevent you from living your life to the fullest.

While the techniques on this e-book let you enhance your degrees of strain, anxiety, and depression, I suggest looking for expert useful useful resource to help push you towards your desires.

There are thousands of books in this venture in the marketplace, so thanks for deciding on this one! "How to Deal with Stress, Depression, and Anxiety" will provide a complete framework and a well-rounded set of system on the manner to understand the motives of pressure, depression, anxiety and the way to triumph over it. Please revel in!

How Your Brain Works
Too many people damage their restoration adventure by means of the use of working within the direction of their minds. They suppose they are capable of stress their brains

into submission, and whilst that doesn't artwork, they experience like failures. When a change you're searching for to make does not stick, it is also as it isn't one your thoughts is used to. As loads as you can want that alternate, your mind will face up to it due to the fact uncommon matters sense unstable to the human brain. The human mind loves styles, and it makes use of the ones patterns to create your internal intellectual programming and perceptions of truth. When you recognize how your brain works, you may use it in your advantage to create new styles and reframe your intellectual u . S . A ..

Your thoughts is a effective stress, and it could art work in outstanding techniques. In dealing with your issues, doubts, and one-of-a-kind terrible emotions, you need to understand how your thoughts functions so you can stop fighting your thoughts and start going for walks with it.

Your Map of Reality

In 1931, scientist and logician Alfred Korzybski set up an essential metaphorical perception collectively alongside along with his statement, "The map isn't the territory." He believed that individuals do now not have absolute facts of truth; as an alternative, they have got a set of beliefs constructed up over the years that have an impact on how they apprehend occasions and situations. People's ideals and views (their map) are not fact itself (the territory). In particular phrases, belief is not reality.

Your thoughts fills gaps in understanding robotically. This technique that at the equal time as you don't recognize a few factor, you subconsciously make an estimation primarily based totally on the records you do recognize. When you revel in fear or sadness, this could be due to a map of reality that complements those thoughts. That worry or disappointment lingers for your mind and can form future selections until you reshape your notion. Your map of truth will commonly be an interpretation, however it could be an interpretation that enables you in vicinity of hurts you. You can trade your map of truth and make it greater productive by means of addressing your thoughts and beliefs and the way they impact your conduct.

Thoughts, Core Beliefs, and Behavior

Beliefs are units of thoughts that humans use to dictate how they'll behave. A belief is some factor you located is a fact. You sense so strongly approximately some element that you're nearly first-rate it's real, irrespective of how well you may show it. You also can have a few doubts on occasion, however, regular, you continuously hold on with those beliefs. Beliefs are attitudes that you fall decrease back on, because of the fact they provide a feel of safety, and they make you experience that certain subjects are constant, this is why some thing that makes you doubt your ideals can be so painful. Your beliefs pressure your subconscious, ordinary behaviors. They turn out to be so ingrained in you that they experience natural and inherently actual.

When you've got were given problem coping with situations or handling emotions, you robotically switch on your beliefs for help without exerting an excessive amount of brainpower. Your ideals assist making a decision morality, and that they assist you decide whether or not or not humans or things are terrible or appropriate. Your entire mind-set uses a compilation of your beliefs to fill in the additives of your truth you could't virtually recognize.

Beliefs are fashioned primarily based on past reviews and the stimuli spherical us. Most human beings's middle beliefs—the maximum driving beliefs they have got—are installation when they're younger youngsters. As they grow old, children commonly mission the beliefs they've been taught as they begin to anticipate more seriously and independently. Nevertheless, many children reaffirm the beliefs they were taught in vicinity of disproving them. As adults, they could venture these ideals and, via way of handling their ideals, they might create a extra suit view of the area that's a more sensible map of truth.

Beliefs may be considerably powerful. For example, believe parents telling their kids that paperclips are volatile. Telling a infant that paperclips are unstable seems stupid. Nevertheless, at the same time as the ones words bypass unchallenged, the child will internalize the message, and they may try to keep away from paperclips, which could prevent their ability to do certain obligations. But as they develop old, the child would possibly possibly task that notion and triumph over the worry of paperclips.

Other beliefs can be more difficult to debunk. For example, if a mom tells her little one that dogs are risky, the child may also additionally moreover turn out to be scared of dogs. This worry may additionally want to preserve into adulthood, because of the truth the child has discovered out to be scared of puppies. Even rational arguments that puppies aren't some aspect to be fearful of can also moreover even though make it hard for that toddler to consider. After all, puppies, in assessment to paperclips, do have the potential to bark and chew. The toddler may be so glad via the use of the perception that it might be tough for them to break from that mind-set.

You may additionally additionally have beliefs that stand for your way and revel in so foundational to who you're that difficult them makes you uncomfortable. Nevertheless, you want to ponder your limiting beliefs.

While mind and beliefs may additionally seem similar, there are a few profound differences among them which you need to famend in case you need to have a whole understanding of the manner your mind and ideals could make or break your intellectual fitness. Thoughts assist to shape your ideals. When you have were given got the same thoughts time and again, they turn out to be ideals. You turn out to be so used to the mind that they come to be ingrained to your subconscious, and it becomes hard to count on that those mind aren't actual. Accordingly, on the identical time as you think negatively, you typically tend to have a more pessimistic outlook.

Not all thoughts are ideals. The thoughts that come and undergo your mind with out repetition by no means become ideals. Beliefs are a crafted from routine questioning. This manner that whilst it could be difficult to break them, you may damage them with the resource of overwriting those horrible mind with first-rate ones, it's a workout that many recuperation methods and techniques cited in this e-book use to reduce strain, tension, and melancholy.

As you've visible with the map of truth, perception shapes our views, and it additionally shapes the way we assume. Your thoughts assemble your beliefs, and your beliefs, in flip, build your revel in of what's actual. Some of your ideals will empower you to are searching out fulfillment and locate happiness, even as others will make the sector look like a darkish and frightening location without a preference. Try to find out the elements of your belief tool that reason you to have terrible responses.

Your belief styles have extremely good electricity to change your life. The smooth act of interrupting terrible concept styles allow you to begin to make adjustments. These changes don't show up in a unmarried day, and deeply entrenched beliefs may additionally even take months or years to debunk in reality, however, while you attention at the concept patterns you want to instill, you begin to question the "truths" you blindly believed.

There is probably a few beliefs you'll want to hold, and people are ones you can assemble upon and use for your gain for the duration of this method. There's no need to take away any belief that's excessive exceptional because such beliefs are individuals who help you expand. However, be honest approximately the ideals which can be hurting you. Many humans try to rationalize fantastic ideals that they revel in psychologically unready to name into question. Open your mind and contemplate, "Is this perception hurting me in covert and manipulative methods?" If you conflict even to pose that question approximately a selected perception, that notion may be a volatile one.

The way you observed isn't a few thing that's out of your control. According to the Massachusetts Institute of Technology (MIT), forty five percent of your each day options are routine, this means that they're a manufactured from your subconscious concept styles and ideals. You pick out what stimuli you feed for your subconscious. When problems or hopelessness start to fill your head, strive announcing to yourself, "The global is a place whole of opportunity and correct matters." While it won't feel like pronouncing that is performing some issue earlier than everything, rewriting your internal monologue can be a effective first step in the direction of increase.

When you apprehend how thoughts and middle beliefs form your behaviors, it will become less complicated to create a direction for increase. You studies that you're in charge of your ideals, and your thoughts can simplest have as masses manipulate over you as you provide them. You may additionally experience helpless in opposition to your terrible mind, however studying to conquer the ones dangerous thoughts and release the energy they've got over you is the quality manner to turn out to be a happier person. The extra you try and keep away from the topics that make you aggravating, harassed, or depressed, the greater worrying, forced, and depressed you'll turn out to be.

Cognitive Distortions

While your mind does its notable to provide you beneficial statistics and create an accurate perception of fact, from time to time it gets a chunk lost seeking to translate what it observes into a realistic perception. Your thoughts likes to make connections, and every so often, it will make connections which might be overly simplified and don't display the nuance in a situation. This is called a cognitive distortion.

Simple speaking, cognitive distortions are falsehoods that your mind persuades you into believing are actual. Cognitive distortions can take pretty some paperwork, but one commonplace example is polarized questioning. When you take delivery of as actual with you studied in polarities, you notice topics as incorrect or proper, suitable or lousy, or win or lose. After you fail at one venture, you can start to assume, "I'll fail each project due to the fact I can't do some thing right." This belief isn't an correct one, however you turn out to be glad it's right because your mind has pinpointed what it thinks is a sample.

The problem with cognitive distortions is that they're regularly shrouded in negativity. They make you anticipate the greater severe, and that they persuade you which you can not do effective matters or that various things are hazardous. Cognitive distortions trade your angle, and they're capable of rapid emerge as dangerous for your popular properly-being. If you trust false messages, it's hard to make peace together together along with your situation or revel in regular. When you enjoy insecure, your intellectual fitness declines, and your doubts start to make it more tough to feature generally. Anxiety might also take hold, and you may sense extra careworn as you attempt to finish obligations. The trouble of your state of affairs may also then motive depression.

Chapter 7: Getting Sober

LIQUID PASSPORTS

The first step within the course of inventing your very very own direction is selecting in which to move. Before you may do this, but, you want to understand wherein you're.

You count on it is probably obvious to absolutely all people who beverages which road they've been travelling down and in which they're now, but addiction is sneaky. Rarely can we be aware the twists and turns along the way due to the fact they'll be so diffused.

The best manner to determine it out is to photo a map of your ingesting adventure. As you have a look at in advance, image the region you're at now with a large crimson arrow pointing to the You Are Here spot. You can begin your sobriety there, within the proper right here and now, or you could maintain your journey to the following stops in advance.

Let's begin with a look at the start wherein, whether or no longer it end up thru peer pressure, experimentation, or sheer stupidity, we took that Very First Drink. Oh wow! That surely didn't flavor so brilliant, huh? But it effective made us experience all fuzzy and happy interior - and we genuinely desired that part! Or we short threw up afterwards and later went yet again till we in the long run observed out to adore it.

Yep. We had to teach ourselves to experience the taste of alcohol. Totally makes us experience like actual geniuses now, proper? Little did we recognize what became prepared up earlier. Had we acknowledged then what we do now, we'd've frozen our steps.

Eventually we crossed into the stylish global of Buzz Chasing. One drink wasn't reducing it any more to get us to that bliss, so we had to upload even greater along the manner. We went from buzz to buzz to buzz, similar to the busy little drinker bees we were. This incredible quest inadvertently led us to a trendy land referred to as Drunk.

Drunk is a completely odd vicinity. Drunk may be especially thrilling or noticeably dramatic, depending on our kingdom of thoughts, how lifestyles is treating us within the interim, and/or who's setting spherical with us at the time. Drunk is a roll of the dice, each bodily and mentally. People also can float there through accident inside the starting, however later begin taking direct flights there intentionally.

We had to take some detours alongside the way to the cities of Puke and Hangovers in advance than we should emerge as greater like real natives of Drunk. And as soon as we determined our manner round drunkenness (did I element out this genius component?) we moreover needed to learn how to maneuver those not so to be had dandy sidekicks referred to as Drama and Regret. Typically, we did so in an "I can cope with it" manner as we began out analyzing the art work of damage manage.

Eventually, countless exercising hours had been invested, as we notion we may additionally want to with the aid of some method get even higher at this ingesting issue. Yep....

Spending an excessive amount of time in the land of Drunk outcomes in a modern-day territory referred to as Tolerance. Much earlier than we expected (or preferred) a few drinks not zipped us alongside to that glad area. Instead, it took many more beverages to seize that buzz and buying even greater rounds with a view to attain that so-called state of drunken bliss. Sure, some red flags may additionally have started out out waving wildly within the ones moments, however we decided out to live with and/or ignore them.

That's while we entered the land of Excuses. Oversleeping, spending extra cash than planned on partying, stupid matters completed on the same time as below the have an effect on, and so forth. Commonly came with a price tag. Instead of proudly proudly owning it, we reassured ourselves with, "This takes region to certainly every person who activities…. Right?" Or probable we pleaded innocence with "What crimson flags? I don't see any purple flags. Nope, no crimson flags spherical right here…." Some people even used them to have amusing.

This factor is in which the paths definitely cut up.

Some humans apprehend whilst to forestall ingesting and (wacky them) achieve this. My head modified into scratched commonly seeking to discern that one out. They see the hazard signs and symptoms and signs and symptoms and reduce themselves off without a doubt or, not less than, reduce manner down. They don't teen themselves thru saying that downing a 12-percentage in a unmarried sitting is a ordinary amount. They're the ones accountable sorts who get their oil checked, ship thank you notes, and mail their taxes in before the very last day. Yeah, them.

Those who hold exploring Drunk on occasion become turning into Happy Hour Alcoholics.

They collect with their friends and/or co-humans for some after elegance or artwork ingesting to "take the threshold off and loosen up" on a ordinary basis. At instances, they even choose to task to Drunk in a set try. This ritual typically takes location among 4 and seven p.M. And frequently magically extends to a abruptly later bedtime. Oops. Of path, the tab totals will upward push after Happy Hour ends however, via that element, they certainly received't care what price they need to pay to benefit admission to Drunk. Your bartender thank you you, truely.

Some pick out out to come to be Weekend Alcoholics as an alternative. They drink in bars, golf equipment, pubs, sports, or in the privacy of their very personal homes. They don't realize they in reality have a problem due to the truth "it's certainly on the weekends", certainly so they hold down this direction till...hmmm...it's not only on the weekends anymore. The bars and liquor shops are magically open throughout the weekdays too. Voila!

Some decide to hop onto the rocky course referred to as Binge Drinking. This is the handiest wherein you get to inform yourself you have to now not have a hassle due to the truth you don't drink every single day. You can't be a actual alcoholic then, proper? Instead, they actually discover themselves having or they locate themselves having twenty.

There's moreover this certainly narrow spot called In Between that everyone gets to discover, where they decide to surrender for a while however magically don't. Instead, they get to experience some sudden and regularly repeated moments of promising God, themselves, and quite a splendid deal absolutely everyone round who can pay interest, that they'll by no means (ever, ever!) ever drink that a good deal all over again. And then they do.

From there, a few pick out to go to extremes and journey down the normal avenue of Daily Drinker. This is in which Binge Drinking leads, however greater out of necessity than choice because the attempting vs. Desiring a drink (aka withdrawals) transition begins. They start to lead cleansing cleaning soap opera lives as debt kicks in due to financing a hungry addiction. The drama is ordinary, both outside and inner. They alienate all people as they become deaf to the sound of demanding voices and that big, pesky, booming one in each of truth.

This is while folks that are in fact addicted will try and adapt. It is what it is and stopping is honestly no a laugh. However, the longer you live in Drunk, the more difficult your frame tries to deal with even massive quantities of what is now essentially poison on your device. That's why a few will inadvertently excursion to that final region that is really called Dead.

There are tremendously unhappy exceptions, but rarely do you ever find out a person deliberately partying to get to Dead. Dead truely form of jumps right out of the timber and surprises individuals who anticipate they'll truly manage their addiction or agree with tomorrow is a much better time to stop. Their bodies surrender, or there's an coincidence, or they pick a combat or…. You get the idea.

Most of you don't forget that eating obtained't kill you. I get that. But I certainly went from "I can take care of it" one night time, as I had 1000 or so nights in advance than, to the subsequent night while my frame very decided "Nope, no longer plenty." I couldn't save you consuming without going into withdrawals.

In that situation you get to do no longer-so-suitable things like having panic attacks, dealing with your very very own mortality, and not having the ability to maintain in smooth such things as a bit of meals or water. Your frame blatantly rejects everything besides the alcohol as your dependancy essentially attempts to kill you.

If you've skilled that thoughts-blowing 2d, exactly what I advocate. Please don't forget getting clinical assist for seizures, extreme dehydration, and/or hallucinations in any other case you could, absolutely, die. Dead, albeit a very eternal solution, is actually not a route.

There's an invisible line amongst that trying to drink and desiring to element, and you don't always figure out in advance of time which you've crossed it. When you're within the land of Addicted, you're in reality too tousled to be purpose.

So, now that we've looked at the map, permit's try the use of desirable judgment instead of emotion for a 2d. You've just taken a observe how to procure right right here, in which you in the interim are, and which way you may be headed. Mark your modern-day spot and think about in which you'd preferably like to transport away your addiction within the again of.

That's all you need to do for now. That's the "homework" for this financial disaster. Ask yourself simply how an extended manner you need to move.

Instead of finishing the journey sincerely, or staying stuck internal a bottle forever, how approximately sorting out this different vicinity called Sobriety at the equal time as you're organized? Contrary to well-known perception, it's no longer a few dark jail full of ordinary desperation for a few other drink. Instead, it's far going to be the whole thing you want it to be due to the fact you are going to be the most effective who designs it.

Plus, you may continuously waft lower back if you hate it, proper? Think about that.

There's a big difference among creating a existence you could simply include vs. Leading one complete of stress and moments you regret. Once you've created the only you need and located out your way spherical Sobriety, you hardly ever locate your self trying to adventure backwards another time. It simply doesn't enjoy sincerely worth it.

Instead, you virtually want to assemble a lakeside cabin and stay.

MAGNIFYING GLASSES

Now that your map is created, the subsequent device you'll need is a magnifying glass.

No one stops to observe the satisfactory print approximately eating when they're inside the middle of dependancy - often because of the truth they don't want to look it or may not even recognize it exists. The massive print, as an alternative, is fairly obvious.

There's been an ongoing industrial for alcohol in our lives. Just take a peek at the people eating within the commercials, suggests and films we see. Look at that glad couple sipping wine through a hearth. Check out that organization of pals downing snap shots and giggling on the bar. Don't neglect approximately approximately those beer-clinking beachgoers promoting liquid happiness with an open invitation to be just like them.

Of route, nobody's shining a highlight on Joe, the under the have an effect on of alcohol in the alley who surely peed at some stage in himself, proper? Poor Joe honestly wasn't hip sufficient to make the cut.

Alcohol is embedded in our history. Note that big-name beer enterprise sponsoring the soccer game you're looking. Behold the classified ads letting us realize that our tour celebrations aren't complete without the sparkling wine to toast each one in all a kind with. And don't neglect the ones circle of relatives BBQ's.

It's been round us in advance than we had been antique sufficient to even understand what it in reality have become and so not unusual that, by the time we do, we view consuming as a general a part of subjects. In a manner, we've been desensitized. Drinking appears so…normal.

Those liquid strings of social bonding can be absolutely considered if you go searching any bar or membership. There's continuously a person sipping "courage" inside the nook and seeking to in shape in. There's that hard guy stopping inside the alley over some detail that wouldn't have even mattered whilst he changed into sober. There's typically someone getting soooo drunk they are able to barely feature and who will become the huge call of a hilarious tale the subsequent morning. "She did whaaa?..."

We're simply free to toss returned some without judgement so long as we give up the car keys as quickly as we skip the prison restrict, right? Absolutely no one will question it or appearance down on it if a person orders a drink. In truth, some might also moreover even begin to marvel about you in case you don't be a part of in on the ritual. Let's have a toast to whichever excuse we've offer you with nowadays. Hooray!

We are all more than welcome, and frequently advocated, to put in writing down down our private permission slips into faux truth. If you purchase the fee price tag, you get to take the enjoy. If you don't like the adventure, properly then, boo. You're genuinely no amusing, are you?

Though we're all privy to exactly in which this journey can lead some of human beings, come what can also moreover society is also ok with that too. Did your buddy have some too many? Oops. Let's try and capture the ones falls and preserve their hair decrease lower back as they spill the contents of that night time time's happiness into the rest room. Very few "pals" will ever prevent to surprise why that they had too many beverages in the first area even though.

It's all a part of the it's-good enough-charade. Since there's no surefire manner to are looking ahead to simply how rapid a person's reached "an excessive amount of" or who's crossed the road into addiction, we anticipate it's all awesome. It'd be first-rate if some type of a buzzer went off to warn you while you've reached your limit, or your skin can also want to start to reveal a weird colour of green to indicate overindulgence, or some bell may ring the minute you've long beyond from informal ingesting to "oh crap you're in trouble now".

Nope. And even then, people are still people. Warning signs or no longer, they're positive to maintain going as it's loads an lousy lot a whole lot much less fun to save you. It's now not like truly each person has to surrender consuming and, receive as actual with me, they gained't. The past has tested stopping doesn't work for society. Alcohol is now not prohibited due to the truth prohibiting it delivered about way more problems than maintaining it prison did. It needed to be normalized.

That's why nobody honestly questions this "ok drug" (yep, we've all been doing pills) in recent times. It's a tool so with out problems appropriate and available that 1/2 of the populace reaches for it on a everyday basis. Of path, doing capsules actually shouldn't be considered regular. If clearly all and sundry round us became tripping out on acid, we'd in all likelihood rethink this concept and we'd honestly take a look at the problem.

Alcohol is trickier than that. A little alcohol seems regular for optimum human beings. A lot of alcohol will become obviously volatile. We usually discover too late that, as soon as the ones tolerance limits get bumped up, the 2 liquids that used to sit down down again someone out are mere stepping-stones to the 5 they'll need later to get humming.

And why will we need that buzz? Because we stay in a worldwide that looks for short fixes. Drinking has lengthy been the correct way to take the brink off our problems, drown those sorrows, and feature amusing the successes. Friends gathering together to drink has emerge as an extended-lasting ritual. Having one or after work is not some thing to word or query.

So, we don't.

The hassle is a few people can persist with that tumbler of wine with dinner and some humans grow to be downing the complete bottle in response to a bad day.

Heaven is aware of that bottle is simple to gain. Unlike pharmaceuticals, you don't need to get a phrase from a clinical physician as a manner to ingest it. Wander proper as lots as the bar and order as many as you need to from the "pharmacist" till they reduce you off. Pop right right right into a liquor keep and you could buy sufficient alcohol from the "company" to throw a celebration. No questions asked, notwithstanding the fact that the ones three instances of beer are satisfactory for your solo weekend of binge gaming. Shhhh….

What's sad is how extra people than ever apprehend how ingesting can cause large problems, but the extensive variety of alcohol related deaths isn't taking location, however up. Big issues generally name for huge interest, however at the identical time because it's a hassle 1/2 of society has been lured into, it's come what may also k to do little to without a doubt remedy it. The evidence is almost screaming at us, however we nonetheless cowl our eyes and ears (los angeles-l. A.-LA, I can't pay interest you) and desire the hassle magically fixes itself.

We, as a collective group of people aka society, were gazing at the act of ingesting through rose-coloured glasses; and we've accomplished so in essential terms inside the call of socializing, break out, income, and blind reputation. Society shades our options about alcohol; and it appears it will hold glorifying the contents of those bottles to the users it permits. The cigarette selling cowboys are prolonged long lengthy beyond now, however alcohol although receives that pinnacle agency time.

Of direction, if society were sincere, we'd prevent performing like consuming is a sensible or practical technique to something the least bit. Even for individuals who don't get addicted.

The bottom line is you had been shown the big print your whole existence. You have been advocated in advance than you even started out eating. You by no means concept alcohol can also additionally effect you for my part in any other case you can have run like hell. Now you're struggling and also you definitely need those bodily and highbrow cravings to vanish so you can reclaim your lifestyles without this proverbial monkey dwelling in your once more.

That monkey will hold on tight for expensive lifestyles until you're so sucked into addiction that it will become an elephant and fills up each room you input. That's while the whispers start ("Is he stumbling, over again?" or "She smells like beer.") as our ears begin burning at domestic, the office or, occasionally, even inside the bar.

Hypocrites.

Though it's outstanding clean to stomp our ft in anger and issue at the arena, we are capable of't. There's hundreds of temptation to play the blame sport proper here. The entire society detail, the those who served as horrible feature fashions, the difficult breaks to your existence....The listing of motives is going on. They're all valid in our minds.

Still, we made the selection to hold – even though we knew matters have been terrible.

In our personal lives, the pals who didn't party a whole lot were changed via those who did. Work or university became a issue to get thru. The financial enterprise account grew emptier because the credit score card ran up. Things we used to care approximately took a backseat to the simplest issue we cared approximately maximum: getting each distinct drink.

We had masses of examples of what no longer to do in our lives. Some folks had the warning tag associated with our thoughts within the form of an alcoholic determine. Some watched consuming pals step away for rehab, excellent to return and begin the cycle over again. Some noticed real death and however stuffed the ones glasses, if most effective absolutely to forget about about.

That's the double-sided sword of addiction: You see it exists and that it's turning into a problem, however you form of don't see it due to the truth the eating shields you. It sees your truth and turns it into high-quality print. It dilutes the reality and disguises itself as a few shape of savior. It makes everything else seem smaller. Including you.

Now's an exceptional time to look closely at those teeny tiny letters you can not want to appearance. The ones that create statements approximately how we must non-public the alternatives we've made. Though you can avoid defensive a magnifying glass over this problem for as long as possible, in the long run it's going to get so big that there might be no desire but to apprehend it's there.

And proper here you are. You've intentionally overlooked your functionality to say the phrases "no thanks" and stored on announcing "positive please" to society, your pals, and your dependancy as a substitute. Stop and consider that for a minute.

Once you bravely admit the reality which you've decided in this, you could empower your self to exchange. You can crack open the door to sobriety.

That's at the same time as ownership shifts far from the dependancy and lower back to you.
NOT ME

Let me will let you comprehend about a famous undertaking some of the "unsober" need to play:
It's called Not Me.

Chapter 8: Bottle Divers

It's tempting to revel in a piece sorry for your self even as you do not forget getting sober. You realize you're no longer the simplest one with this dependancy trouble, however you revel in like come what may additionally your state of affairs is more tough. You think about telling someone, but you experience find it irresistible's going to be all weird and awkward in case you do.

The worst element is you have got got a gut feeling that pretty some people already apprehend. Every appearance on your direction seems like it's loaded with disdain, pity, anger, disappointment, or judgement. It's as if a massive highlight is following you everywhere you're, and also you've end up a suspect in some crime.

That makes you revel in demanding and/or irritated. Who are they to appearance down on you? It's your life, not theirs! So, you make a decision to vent a hint and take a look at the waters with people who may also recognize and sympathize: your eating friends. Even then it feels regular to even talk it.

They will faux to recognize. They will surely sympathize. They will decrease back up your anger with statements about how every body should honestly mind their very personal business employer and tell you now not to care. They love you and could fortuitously be part of you in the subsequent spherical, that is truly imagined to take the strain off.

Eventually, a few drinks later, you revel in higher approximately subjects. These are your real pals. They have your lower returned. They beneficial useful resource you. They understand you.

Of direction they do given some of them are probable fellow applicants for sobriety. Here's a clue: If a person talks about a hassle that they'll be consuming too much, the regular response isn't always to speak you out of that wondering.

The reply from someone who in reality offers a damn is "How can I help?".

That's whilst your head starts offevolved offevolved to fill with questions on the ones humans you celebration with. Do they've got addiction troubles too? How come some of them don't seem to have any consequences for their eating and can keep on a regular lifestyles? Why didn't actually every person else turn out to be on this liquid prison? Were you weaker than them? Were you too silly to word the symptoms and symptoms and symptoms and signs and symptoms? Shouldn't you've got were given recognised higher?

Nope, nope, and nope. There is honestly nothing incorrect with you. You aren't at all "bizarre", and also you possibly did not something to "deserve" this problem. You were sincerely greater susceptible to the tug of addiction. There's an entire army of addicts to be had asking those particular subjects. You're surely ultimately starting to evoke.

Along the twisted road of our addictions, we've been granted the possibility to meet a massive type of human beings - maximum of them with out a hassle located in golf equipment, after hours occasions, and bars. It's easy that addiction welcomes surely anyone with open hands, regardless of profits, pores and skin color, sexual choice, age, faith, or intelligence stage. The more the merrier! You are one in all many, many more.

Back as soon as I scouted, booked, and wrote bios for artists in the track agency, I started to appearance addiction rearing its ugly head more often. From the poorest character in the alley at the back of the stadium to the insanely wealthy one performing at the degree earlier than masses, the faces of addiction went from one cease of the spectrum to the opportunity. The parallels were great at times.

The month I prevent drinking, I witnessed a totally famous (millions of statistics presented) singer stumbling round behind the curtain as he awaited his subsequent recuperation and a homeless woman in a detox phoning a friend to hold her a bottle even as she have been given out. They each had the best identical dependancy issues, but every had particular "connections", allow's don't forget?

The latter became seen inside the course of my stint in an orange uniform furnished by means of the usage of the detox I introduced myself to for twenty-four hours to get past my withdrawal seizures. Yes, it turn out to be run like a jail and virtually felt like one. They have been pretty surprised after I checked myself in vs. Being dragged in by way of the cops. They had been moreover greatly surprised that my heart become nonetheless beating after my breathalyzer check results.

Although my mind emerge as spinning from dehydration, I brief became curious about the collection of "site visitors" sharing this region with me. Some of the captives have been the stereotypical bums at the corner who'd positioned a free bed and meal charge tag via intentional misbehaving. I predicted to peer the ones faces. It changed into humans who have been added in unwillingly that surprised me and held my interest.

These were all very "regular" humans, yet that that they had partied sufficient to be tossed in to dry out and examine their lesson. The exclusive our our bodies within the beds have been as numerous as the ones around us on any metropolis street. There were pilots and doctors and housewives and CEO's and plumbers and...the list is lengthy. Regardless of our backgrounds, I have come to be surrounded through people absolutely as screwed up as I modified into. We were addicts who'd allowed consuming to influence us to some extent wherein each person shared this unhappy reality of assigned beds and canned lectures from the counselors.

It come to be then that I started out to consult them, and myself, as Bottle Divers. To positioned it clearly, each human beings became still seeking out solutions internal of a bottle of alcohol. You'd think the big piles of empty ones within the lower back of us might have been a clue however...a few people simply don't answer their wake-up calls till they need to.

Sometimes we see Bottle Divers at the information. We've watched the memories on a underneath the have an effect on of alcohol driver killing a person or family and/or themselves, right? I've moreover visible the fine approximately the university girl who became dropped off with the resource of "friends" one night time after partying. She fell asleep on the incorrect porch in sub-0 temperatures and ended up dropping most of her palms and ft. The last issue she had tweeted about have grow to be how she turn out to be downing her tenth shot of tequila.

We've moreover heard the tales about the celebrity Bottle Divers who with the aid of twist of destiny drank themselves to loss of lifestyles. Or they don't end and have become a running shaggy dog tale as an alternative. When you look lower returned on the statistics of the superb musicians, artists, actors, and writers, you'll spot a direction of dependancy following behind loads of them. These sorts typically generally generally tend to swim in an ocean of sensitivity. They get without trouble overwhelmed with the resource in their emotions without their "numbing oil" to calm them. They fail to offer without a few aspect to set that creativity loose.

www.ingramcontent.com/pod-product-compliance
Lightning Source LLC
Chambersburg PA
CBHW050409120526
44590CB00015B/1897